FOREWARD

Modern Hypnosis With Today's Science and Technology

The Pope approved Hypnosis in 1956
The Roman Catholic Church banned Hypnotism until the mid-20th century when, in 1956, Pope Pius XII gave his approval of Hypnosis. He stated that the use of Hypnosis by health care professionals for diagnosis and treatment is permitted.

The acceptance of Modern Hypnosis gained significant momentum when that scientifically and morally conservative institution, the Catholic Church, with its well known teachings regarding free will and personal accountability recognized the efficacy of Modern Hypnosis.

The US government was not far behind following the experiences of the Korean conflict and in the late 50's conducted extensive research in various forms of Hypnosis and related fields. There was a significant increase in academic interest and published studies starting in the 90's.

Today, contemporary Behavioral psychology, Biology, Medical diagnostic Imagery and even consumer oriented Technology are all producing insights understanding and extraordinary enhancements to this anciently recognized phenomenon.

Today, our Science and Technology is moving at a increasingly rapid rate making any specific concepts or implementations found in this manual, eligible for replacement or improvement.

The Mission of this Manual is to produce a basic understanding of Hypnosis, and proven implementation of procedures with suggested equipment and software leading to personal or professional enhancement and optionally, credible certification as a Hypnotist.

Modern Hypnosis

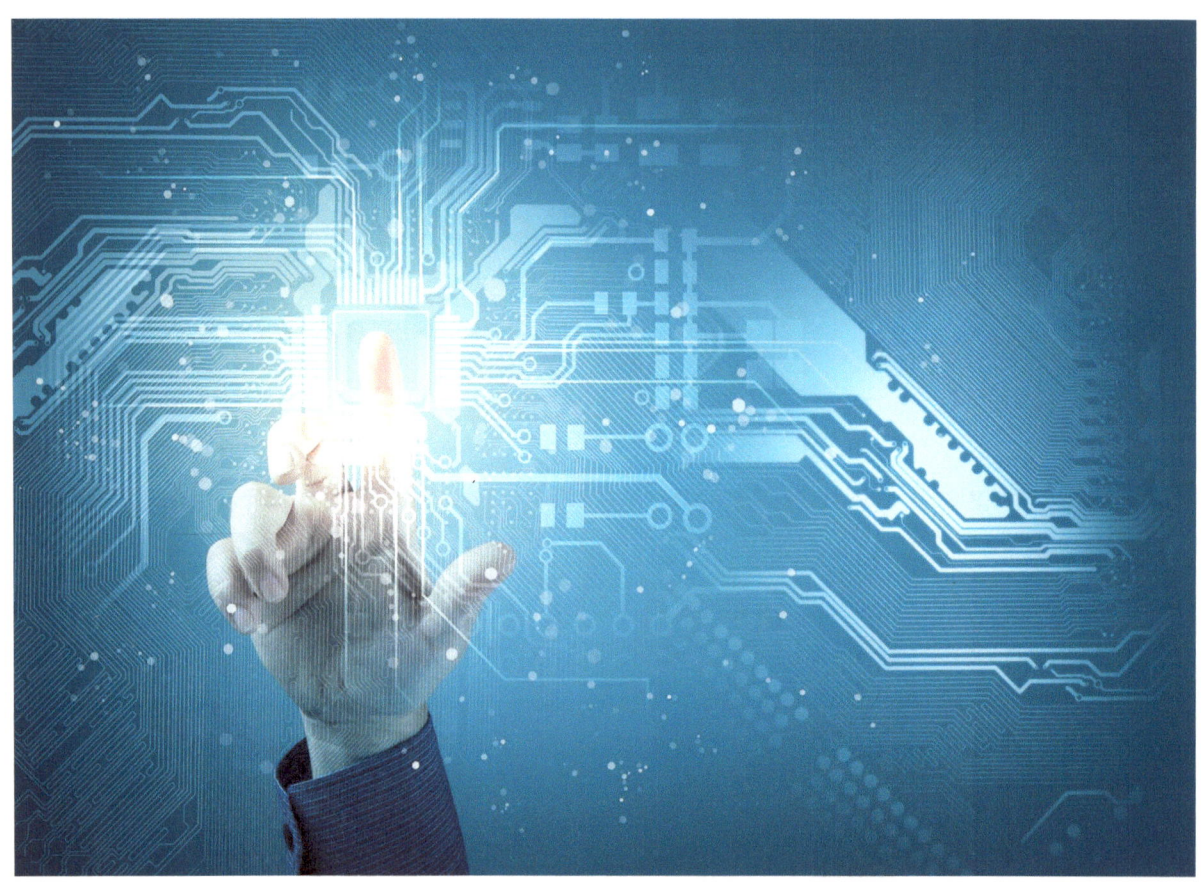

Palm Beach Hypnosis Institute(PBHI)
Palm Beach Florida
Authorized and Certified by the Florida Holistics Institute

US Definition of Hypnotherapist

The U.S. (Department of Labor) Directory of Occupational Titles (D.O.T. 079.157.010) supplies the following definition:

"Hypnotherapist – Induces hypnotic state in client to increase motivation or alter behavior pattern through hypnosis. Consults with client to determine the nature of problem. Prepares client to enter hypnotic states by explaining how hypnosis works and what client will experience. Tests subject to determine degrees of physical and emotional suggestibility. Induces hypnotic state in client using individualized methods and techniques of hypnosis based on interpretation of test results and analysis of client's problem. May train client in self-hypnosis conditioning.

Australia

Professional hypnotherapy, Hypnotherapist or clinical Hypnotherapists not government-regulated in Australia.

In 1996, as a result of a three-year research project led by Lindsay B. Yeates, the Australian Hypnotherapists' Association[40] (founded in 1949), the oldest hypnotism-oriented professional organization in Australia, instituted a peer-group accreditation system for full-time Australian professional Hypnotherapists, the first of its kind in the world, which "accredit[ed] specific individuals on the basis of their actual demonstrated knowledge and clinical performance; instead of approving particular "courses" or approving particular "teaching institutions"" (Yeates, 1996, p.iv; 1999, p.xiv). [41]The system was further revised in 1999.[42]

Hypnotherapy in the United Kingdom

Hypnotherapy is currently unregulated in the UK. However, following recommendations made by the House of Lords Select Committee on Science and Technology (1999), discussions have taken place into the voluntary self-regulation (VSR) of hypnotherapy. In 2002, the Department for Education and Skills developed National Occupational Standards for hypnotherapy linked to National Vocational Qualification based on National Qualifications Framework under The Qualifications and Curriculum Authority. And thus hypnotherapy was approved as a stand-alone therapy in UK. There are now many training schools which claim that their qualifications are "nationally recognized" or "conform to national occupational standards" but there is no way of independently verifying this. _From Wikipedia, the free encyclopedia_

To enhance your learning Experience We Recommend that before reading any further, FIRST take the self administered test on PG 107

The learning objectives of This Course
:

The students will understand Modern, Ethical, State of the art Hypnosis and the results of applied research in this discipline. The student will learn to assess a client so as to determine the most effective induction method, The student will then, be able to exploit recent advances in Science and Technology, create beneficial suggestions, evaluate the depth of the client's Hypnotic Trance, and demonstrate in situ to the examiner the successful induction of a Hypnotic Trance.

The In Clinic, Basic, Hypnosis Course is composed of Lecture, Discussion, and actual practice including applied, state of the art hardware technology and software.

This in Clinic course will take 2weeks, (8 days in class), Monday through Thursday, 9 to 1, reinforced with approximately 25 hours of home study and assignments Plus 1 day of written and oral Exams followed by the Student's in situ qualifying demonstrations.

Alternatively: *For Certification as a result of self study using this manual, follow the instructions in the last chapter.*

Basic course – (1 on 1, in Clinic)

You will find this This basic course is ideally suited as a foundation to either Advanced Certification and the professional practice of Hypnotherapy or to increase the modalities available in your existing professional practice.

Many individuals who have taken this course have learned how to instill in themselves significant positive changes and implemented the insights, techniques and practices found in modern ethical Hypnosis, to permanently enhance their lives as well as their Clients

The In Clinic course prerequisites are:

The student's affirmation that he or she has sufficient command of English as a spoken and written language, the ability to understand and implement the study material and instruction which they will be required to demonstrate continuously throughout the course by demonstrations, oral and written examination by the instructor.

If at any time during the In Clinic Course, *The student cannot continue*, or The instructor determines that the student is *not* meeting the expected requirements *or fails* the final oral written or demonstration of Hypnosis, the Palm Beach Institute of Hypnosis will offer to the student, at the option of The Director,

1. A refund of 50% of the *fees* collected

2. Re-examination for certification 30 days later.

Course material
The PBHI Basic course, student manual

Total Required Hours :

Actual Classroom……………………………… ……………….32 hrs

Required home study and written assignments…………. 25 hrs

Examiner administered, oral interview, written 51 Question Test, and Student's demonstration of a complete successful Hypnotic induction……………………..5 hrs
Total…………………..62 hrs

Suggested supplemental study

The Edinburgh Lectures on Mental Science by.............................Thomas Troward
Hypnosis and Self Hypnosis by ....Prof.Kurt Tepperwein
Patterns of the Hypnotic Techniques by...Dr.Milton H. Erickson,MD
Uncommon Therapy by... Jay Haley
Mindfulness and Hypnosis by... W.W. Norton
Computer Design and Brain Structure By...H.L.Silvia MCH PhD
Hypnosis and the Power of Positive thinking by ....Dr. D.A. Brady
Articles and Lectures By..Gil Scott Fitzgerald-Master Hypnotist

Assessment
Assessment will be accomplished in multiple modes:

Daily written Q and A sheets related to previous, class instructions discussions and homework assignments some of which will include the creation of, original induction and suggestion scripts

Individual student demonstrations of of Hypnosis sessions and written evaluation of the demonstrations by the instructor.

An in situ demonstration to the examiner of a successful induction

The final written exam

Upon successful completion of the course The participants will be Eligible for Certification application at the Florida Holistics Institute

Modern Hypnosis
Student Manual

TABLE OF CONTENTS

Chapter One..page 10

The History of Hypnosis..11
Introduction To Hypnosis...The Hypnotic state.............................14
What Hypnosis can accomplish..16
Specific Applications for Hypnotists and Hypnotherapists..................17
Hypnosis for Addictions...21

Logical-Ethical Limitations..23
A Success story...27
Contemporary Memory Science..28

Chapter Two..page 33

Depth levels of Hypnosis..34
Level Testing..37
Stages in a Hypnotherapy session..39
Rapport,..40
MODELING, MIRRORING AND PACING......................................42
Recognition of various Personalities...45
Subliminal Messaging..44
Suggestibility 47
CAUTIONS..54

Chapter Three...Implementing Today's Technology.............page 59
The Session..60
Computer Mechanical and audio visual Aids...............................61
Inductions..63
Convincers..67
Deepening Techniques..68
Hypnotic suggestions..71
Scripts...75
Reinforcement...73
Understanding The Freedom from Nicotine series......................85
The PBHI Nicotine Script...87
Science and Technology...100

Chapter Four .... page 101

Self – Hypnosis..102
Auto-suggestion...105
Self-Reinforcement Script #1..106
Self-Reinforcement Script #2..107

Chapter Five.. page 108

Analgesia and Anesthesia...109
Maintaining anesthesia..109
Hypnosis with Local or General Chemical Anesthesia...........110
Controlling Bleeding..111
You are almost ready...112
Your First Appointment...113
Conclusion..114
Recommended Equipment and Environment......................115
Software,..116

The Self administered course test......................................118
Exam Key...121

Appendix..124

CHAPTER ONE *The Hypnotic state*

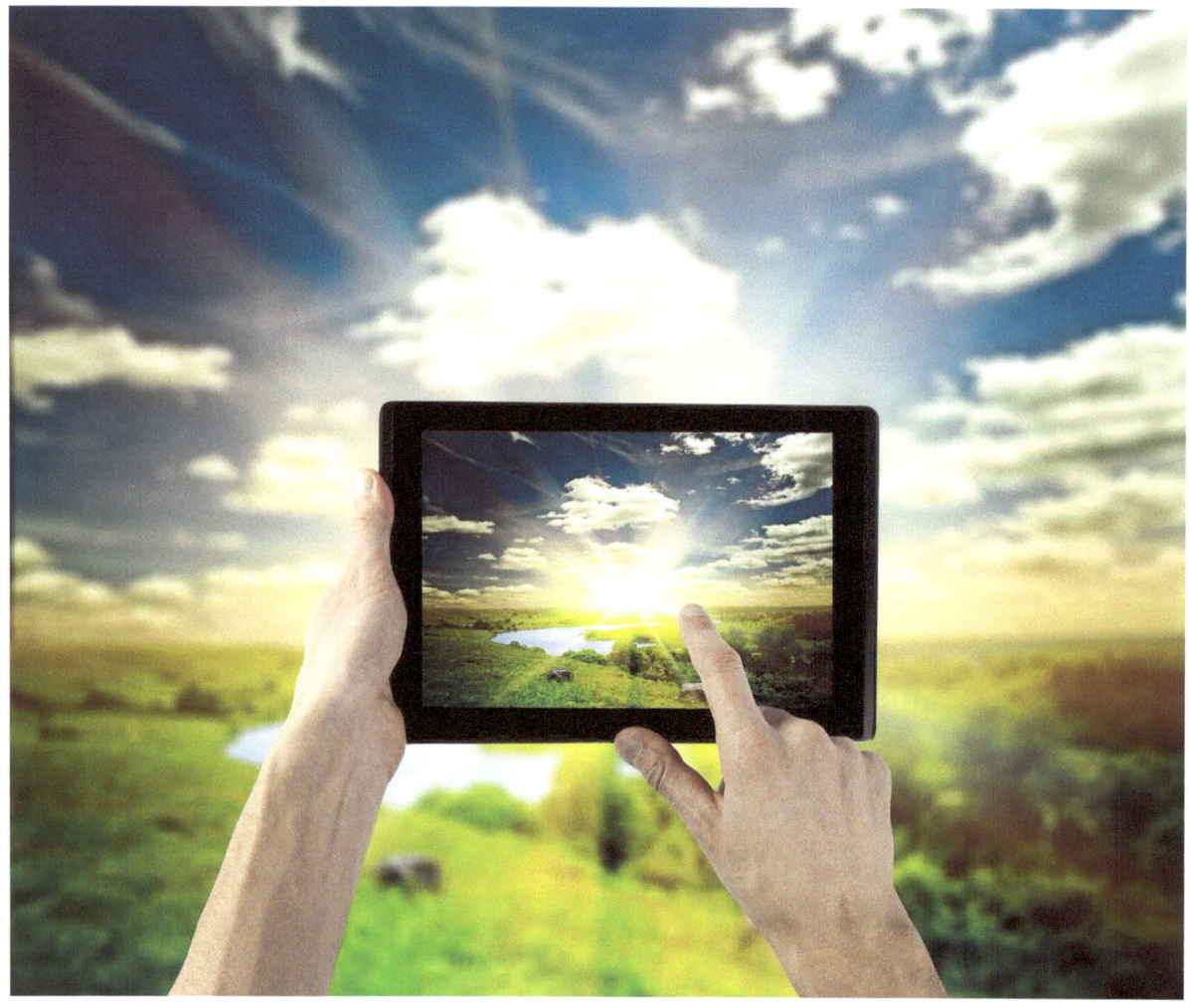

  People going into trance to heal themselves or to retrieve information has been documented throughout human history. Four thousand years before Christ, the Sumerians, according to well preserved cuneiform characters found in the countries bordering the Euphrates and Tigris describe certain methods still in use today. Useful recorded techniques of Hypnosis date back to the 1700's, however, at that time, the human mind and the actual effect of Hypnosis was not scientifically as well understood as it is now.

A BRIEF HISTORY OF HYPNOSIS

References to apparent Hypnotic states are seen in documents over 3500 years old. The priests of ancient Egypt would put patients to "sleep" until health was restored. Those who have read Jean Auel's fictional but well-researched book, "Clan Of The Cave Bear," will remember accounts of magic, healing, inherited memories and revelations performed or created by the "Mog-urs" and "medicine women" of prehistoric clans. Such experiences, plus other historical accounts of healing "sleep" indicate that Hypnotic states were involved.

The more modern era of Hypnosis started with an Austrian physician named Franz Mesmer. Mesmer became convinced that he had a special magnetic field within himself that could connect with the magnetic field of his patients. Complicated and impressive magnetic devices added to his mystique and notoriety. Mesmer performed many apparent cures, often accompanying the sessions with a musical instrument developed by one of his contemporaries, Benjamin Franklin, called the Glass Armonica. A series of spinning crystal bowls on a spindle that, when touched a moistened finger, produced pure musical tones. One of Mesmer's patients, Wolfgang Amadeus Mozart, wrote several compositions especially for the Glass Armonica. When Benjamin Franklin was in France he was asked to participate in an investigation of Mesmer. Mesmer's theory of "animal magnetism" was debunked and he was deemed a fraud which gave Hypnotism a reverse spin into the world of the occult, strengthening many of the false assumptions that have remained until today. Although Mesmer's explanation of how Hypnosis works is considered inaccurate by today's standards, the phenomenon is nonetheless genuine.

Medical interest and acceptance expanded following World War II when the use of Hypnosis proved especially helpful to surviving battlefield casualties suffering from shock, injury, battle fatigue and various psychological disorders. As understanding increased, Hypnosis began to be recognized as an important addition to various medical fields.

It was later demonstrated that Hypnosis could be an important tool in dealing with habits and addictions – both mental and physical

The ascent to respectability began a little more than 30 years ago, when psychologist *Ernest Hilgard*, Ph.D., a former president of the American Psychological Association, set up the Laboratory of Hypnosis Research at Stanford University. At about the same time, psychiatrist *Martin Orne,* M.D., of Harvard and psychologist T. X. Barber, Ph.D., of the Medfield Foundation, pioneered Hypnosis research at their respective organizations. Since then, dozens of research programs on Hypnosis have sprung to life in universities and medical schools in the United States, Canada, Europe, and Australia.

The Technical Services Staff, a part of the Directorate of Science & Technology of the United States Central Intelligence Agency, In the 1950s and early 1960s researched, investigated, and experimented in the use of drugs, chemicals, Hypnosis, and isolation to extract information during interrogation, as well as to make it easier for American captives to resist interrogation.

…..**Psychologists, Theories and Practices:**

…..Freudian psychiatrists *proposed* that Hypnotism involved a close personal relationship between subject who had a "sick" need to be dominated and Hypnotist who had a sick need to "dominate". Later, psychoanalysts incorporated Hypnosis as a treatment modality with their own client-centered , inductions.

James Braid (1785-1860), a British doctor, used eye fixation on objects to induce hypnosis, and gave us the name Hypnosis, (Greek for sleep). He tried later to change the name, but was unsuccessful. He performed thousands of operations using only personally induced Hypnosis.

John Elliotson (1791-1868), a professor of surgery at the University College in London and the inventor of the stethoscope, used Hypnosis for painless surgery and for treating mental disorders.

James Esdalie (1808-1859): Doctor who practiced in India performed surgery with Hypnosis for anesthesia. Note:Hypnosis has been known to be used as anesthesia during eye surgery in India.

Jean Charcot (1825-1893) and Hippolyte Bernheim (1837-1919): French neurologists, first feuded for many years,then collaborated, which led to development of new Nancy School, utilizing suggestions. Many Modern Hypnotists follow this school.

Sigmund Freud (1856-1939): Freud studied under both Charcot and Bernheim. Freud used Hypnosis for a while until he switched to Free Association where the patient does most of the talking. Freud tried to discredit Hypnosis until he was very old. Setting Hypnosis back 70 years. Freud eventually agreed that it was a good method, but that he was not good at it. .

Emile Coue (1857-1926): His technique called "Conscious Auto suggestion, Wrote the most famous positive suggestion of recorded history; it is now being used by members of Alcoholics Anonymous throughout the world.
"Everyday in every way, I'm getting better and better".

Milton Erickson,M.D (1901-1980). Was paralyzed by polio at age 14 and used self-Hypnosis to overcome the illness. Once recovered, he devoted his life to helping others use Hypnosis. The vast majority of Hypnotists today are trained with the teachings of Dr. Erickson. -

The British Medical Association in 1892 ,endorsed the therapeutic use of Hypnosis
Johannes Schultz Adapted techniques and concepts of Yoga and Meditation,and named his system of Auto Hypnosis Autogenic Training. *The Pope* approved Hypnosis in 1956

The Roman Catholic Church banned Hypnotism until the mid-20th century when, in 1956, Pope Pius XII gave his approval of Hypnosis. He stated that the use of Hypnosis by health care professionals for diagnosis and treatment is permitted.

The *Phenomena of Hypnosis*

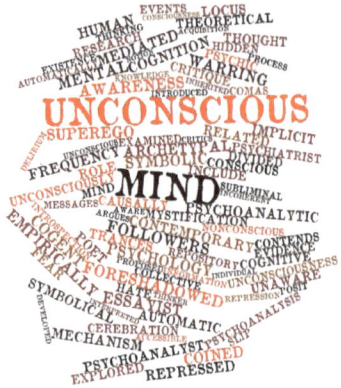

Hypnosis is now so scientifically documented as to render any contrary discussion of its credibility as superfluous. Our responsibility today is the ethical exploitation of this valuable human capability.

The Trance State is actually commonplace. Our minds often depart conscious awareness; For instance, while driving your car, you may realize that while driving long distances, quite a few miles had passed while you were unaware and in a deep daydream, or while performing a repetitive task such as exercising when we lose the count. These moments are a state very close to Hypnosis however Hypnosis is better described than defined. It is often considered a slightly altered state of consciousness, featuring "selective perception"; a process in which the subject chooses to see only what is relevant to the task, blotting out everything else. Hypnosis involves guided concentration. The guidance, however, may be provided by a Hypnotist

A Hypnotherapist will reinforce and expand this state inducing the first level or Alpha state of *total* relaxation, and maintain that brief sense of peace and release we all experience in that instant before we lapse into sleep. The Professional Hypnotherapist will expertly establish and maintain this state, wherein the subconscious mind, will ignore the conscious critical state, and store beneficial information or in the case of self-Hypnosis, by the individual . Self-Hypnosis, which can be taught by a master- Hypnotist to virtually any client, can provide the recipient with a lifetime of benefit.

It is important to note that the *unconscious* mind does not differentiate between fact and fiction. 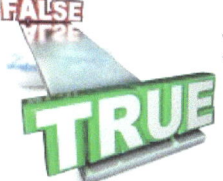 It accepts information and responses as "Data" to be accessed by the conscious or operating function of our minds so that later, in a normal conscious state, the conscious mind will tend to automatically respond with previously determined, benign behavioral responses based on this newly stored information. The effect of a single session seldom lasts more than 48 hours.

The effect and persistency of the suggestions will become stronger with each induction. Subsequent sessions of Hypnosis can be identified as "Classical Conditioning".

Multiple sessions, in the Hypnotic state of susceptibility, will significantly enhance the newly incorporated changes and information until they become *permanent.*

Recording reinforcement or induction sessions for the client to use in their smart phones or mp3 players on a daily basis can both significantly enhance the in person experience and reduce the necessity for multiple sessions...

Many of your clients will appreciate this..

What can Hypnosis accomplish ?

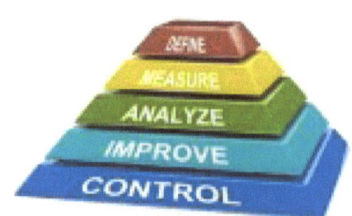

Following World War II, when the use of Hypnosis proved especially helpful to surviving battlefield casualties suffering from shock, injury, battle fatigue and various psychological disorders, experience enhanced its credibility and Hypnosis began to be recognized as an important addition to various medical fields. It has also been demonstrated that Hypnosis could be an important tool in dealing with habits and addictions – both mental and physical.

Hypnotherapy can be described as a way of inculcating positive thinking. Far from being the occult image presented by Mesmer, modern Hypnosis can be a powerful tool to realize positive change in our every day lives.

If a person is desirous a beneficial change in behavior, situational response or attitude then Hypnosis can be the answer. Issues can range from physical fitness to sales performance to Public speaking or even dealing with broken relationships.

Many famous people have used Hypnosis, including Mozart, Frederick Chopin, Thomas Edison, Certain professional golfers, Henry Ford, Winston Churchill and Albert Einstein

Some types of Hypnosis are known as:
Progressive Relaxation
Anodyne Imagery tm
Neuro-linguistic programming(NLP), Pain Management, Guided imagery, Painless Childbirth, and EDMR. (There are Many Others)

Applications:

The possible uses for Hypnosis are only limited by the client's Motivation. As a Hypnotist you can Make no *Medical* claims...but when you can work with enlightened medical and other professionals the results can be significant.

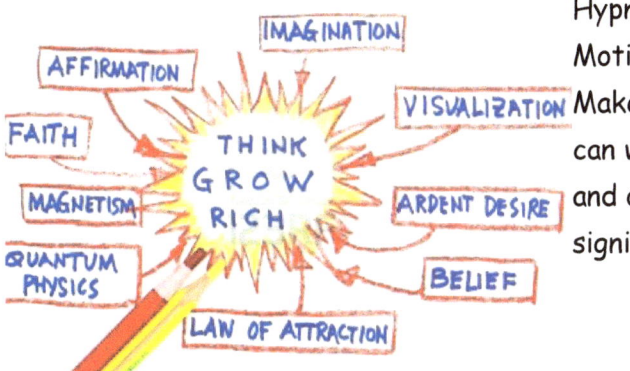

Self Improvement – Increasing athletic performance, memory, psychic skills, public speaking, study skills, self esteem, motivation, self awareness, people skills, time management focus and intense concentration

Undesirable Habits--Stop: stuttering, thumb sucking, bed wetting, worrying, procrastinating, nail biting, obsessive-compulsive behavior

smoking 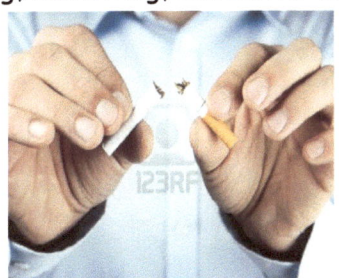 , food cravings. Attitude control,

Replace undesirable tendencies, negative thinking and habits with beneficial behavior

Fears and Phobias 16859977

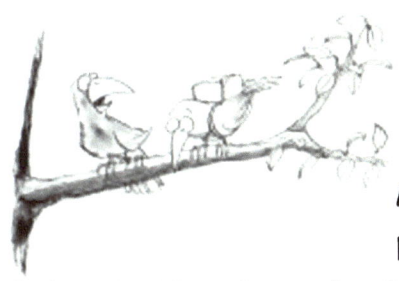

Most subjects can Eliminate fear of: closed-in places, public places, flying, water, or other objects or situations.

"Let's try it without the parachute."

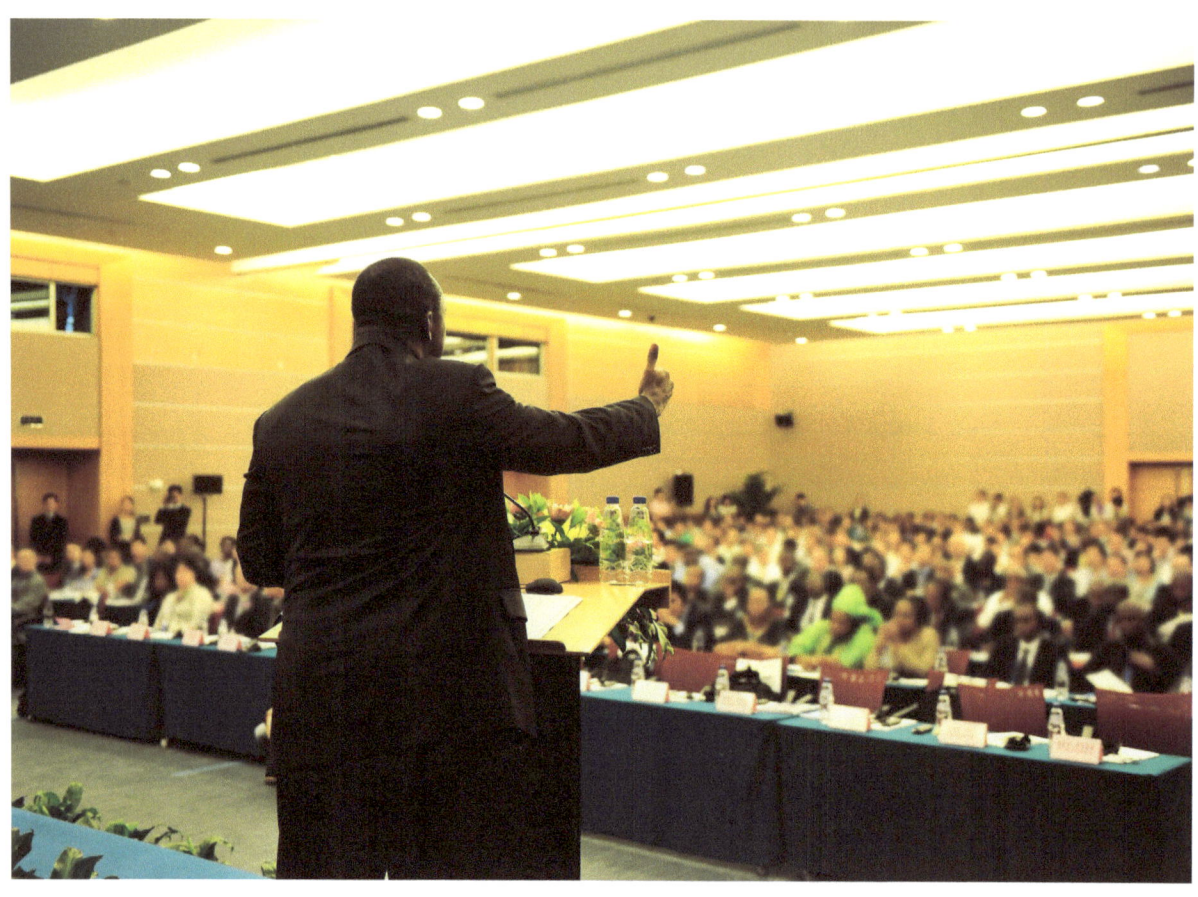

Hypnosis can **Improve or strengthen abilities** in: sales ,Public Speaking Math, Networking or attracting successful Relationships, by projecting positive subliminal visual and audio characteristics

Stress Reduction.....

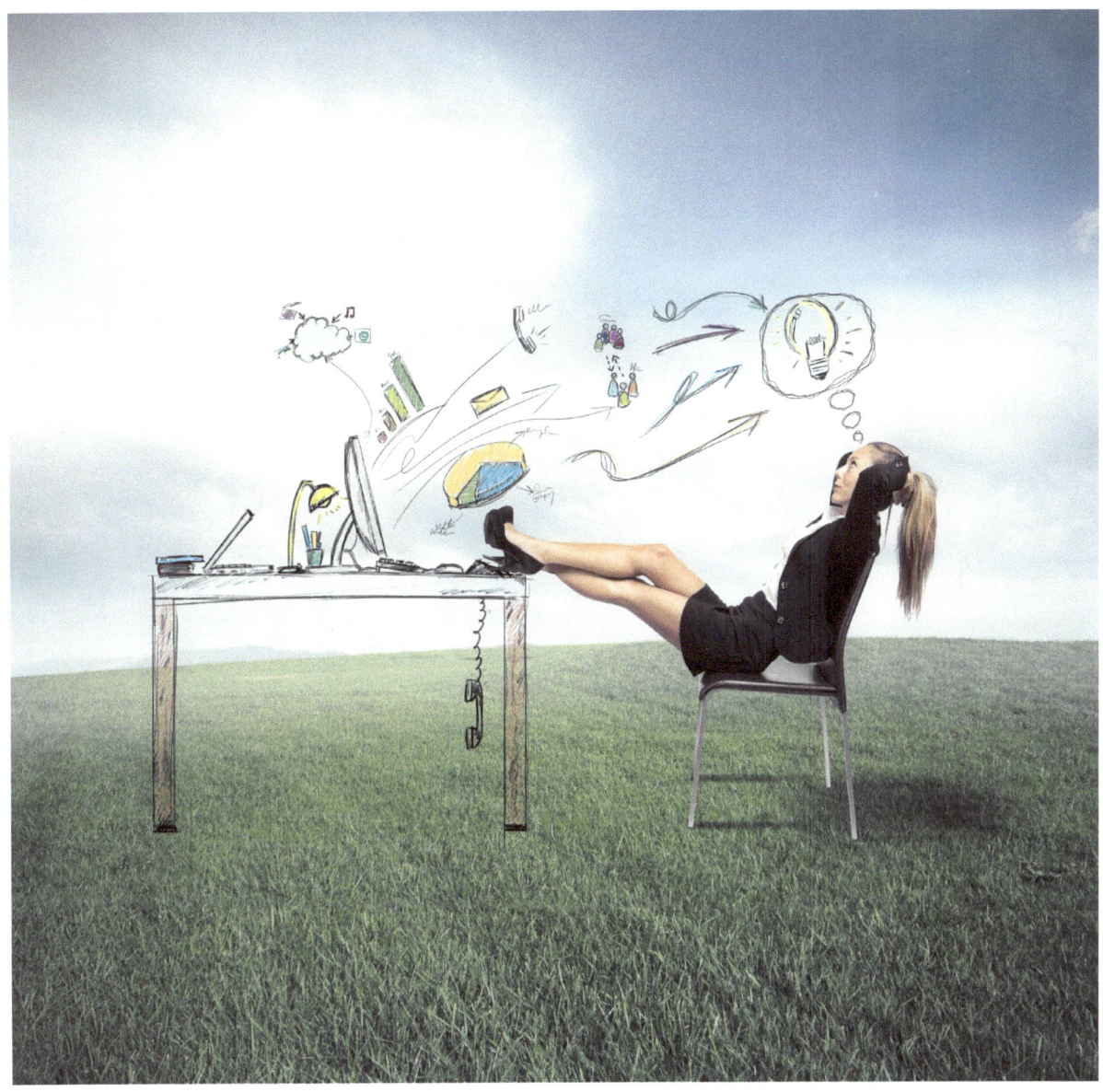

Chemical free total relaxation.

Physical Changes-- Overcoming or Managing Disease, Headaches, and

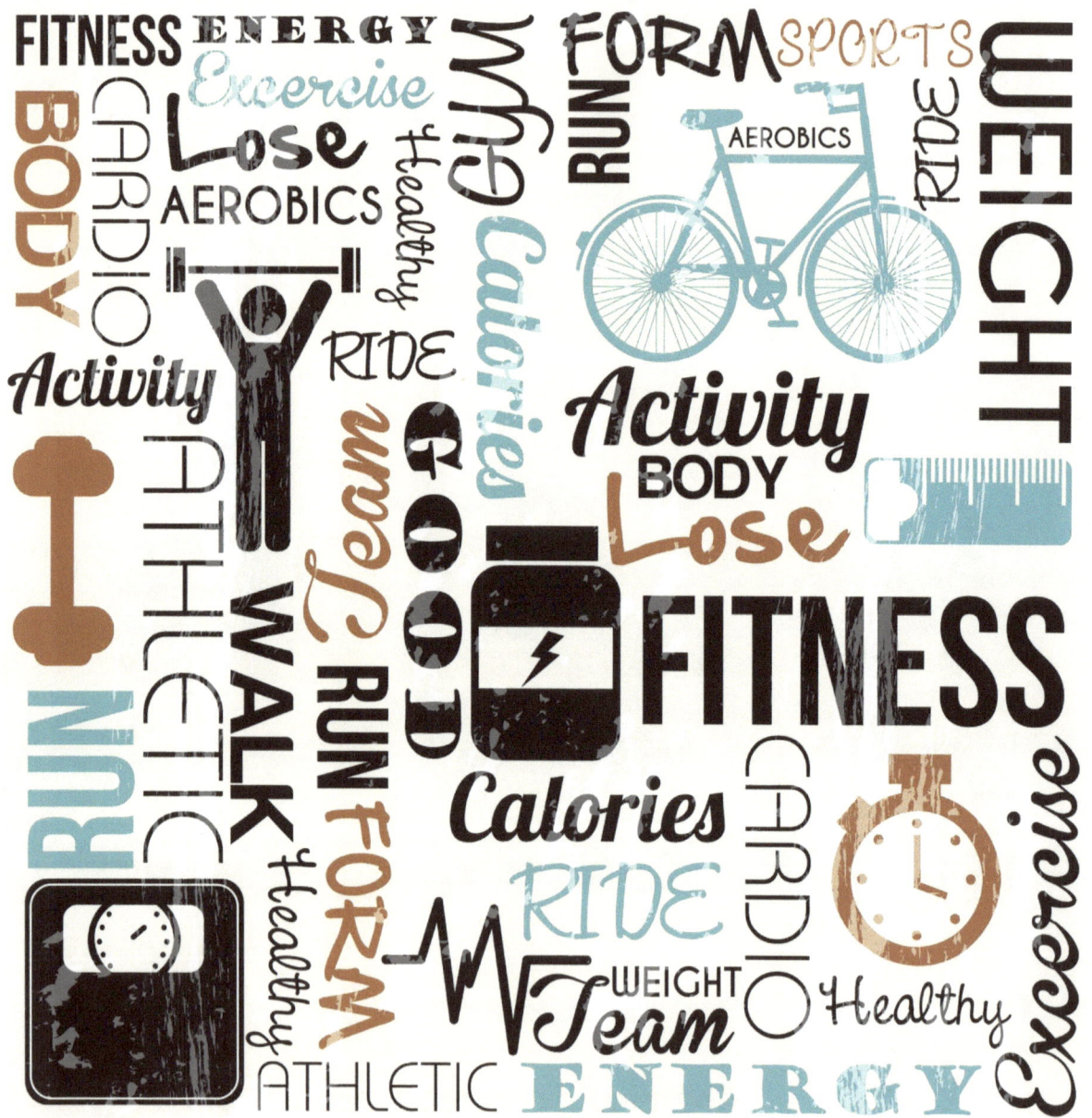

Hypnotherapy is also a very effective method for Chronic Pain, Management :

Hypnosis for Addictions

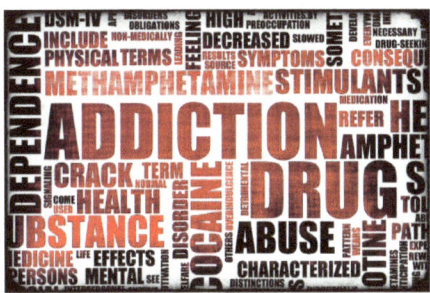

Treatment For any addictive or habitual problem can be effectively reinforced with Hypnosis,

Even a chemical dependence But ……………!

Medical oversight and treatment is essential during the physical withdrawal period as this process can incur life threatening symptoms!

First each person needs to be clean and sober before initiating

Hypnotherapy

Check your local and state licensing requirements. In some states, one must have a specific license to perform Hypno"therapy"

Many studies show that using Hypnotherapy in addition to Twelve Step Programs results in up to 87 percent continued success. Hypnotherapy provides individualized and specific reprogramming which can insure long term relief. The Hypnotist is able to replace old habits with new and healthier ways to relax and unwind. Hypnotherapy is safe, reliable and quick. It helps the addict through the physical and emotional post detoxification discomfort while helping them deal with the aparently new feelings

It is the missing piece of the puzzle.

Addicts Quit with Hypnosis

From a comparative study of hypnotherapy and psychotherapy in the treatment of methadone addicts.
Manganiello AJ.
American Journal of Clinical Hypnosis 1984; 26(4): 273-9.

"94 Percent Remained Narcotic Free with Hypnosis

Significant differences were found on all measures. The experimental group had significantly less discomfort and illicit drug use, and a significantly greater amount of cessation. At the six month follow up, 94 percent of the subjects in the experimental group who had achieved cessation remained narcotic free."

"Although Hypnosis may not be a stand-alone treatment but when it is expertly combined with other therapies, such as a 12-step program, Hypnosis can be an extremely effective approach." - **Psychology Today, 9/96**

Logical-Ethical Limitations

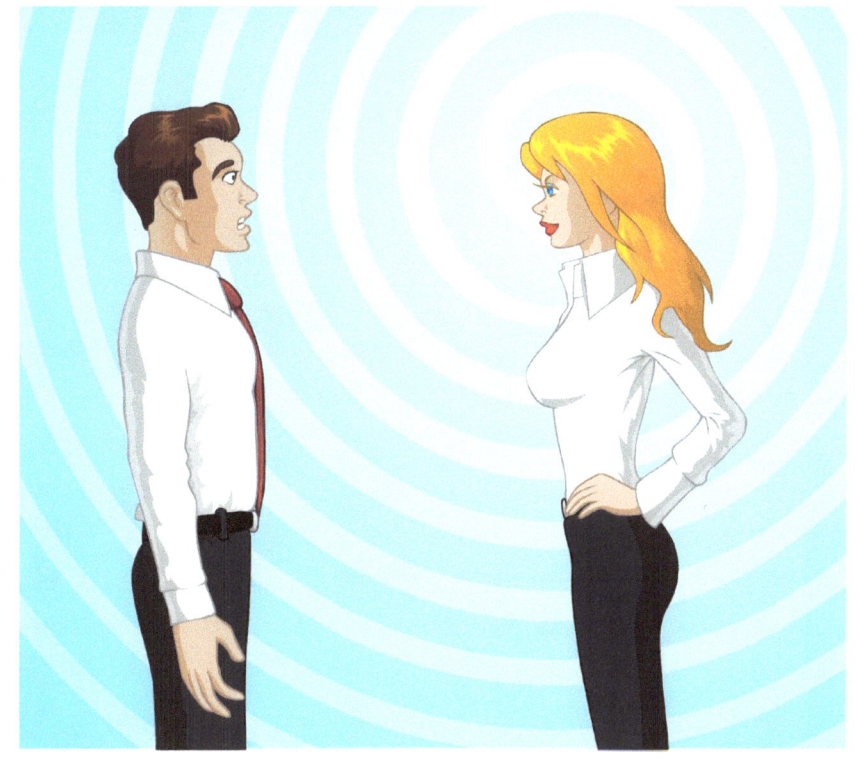

Even though Hypnosis is effective and completely safe, few procedures are less understood, or more plagued by misconceptions and misunderstandings.

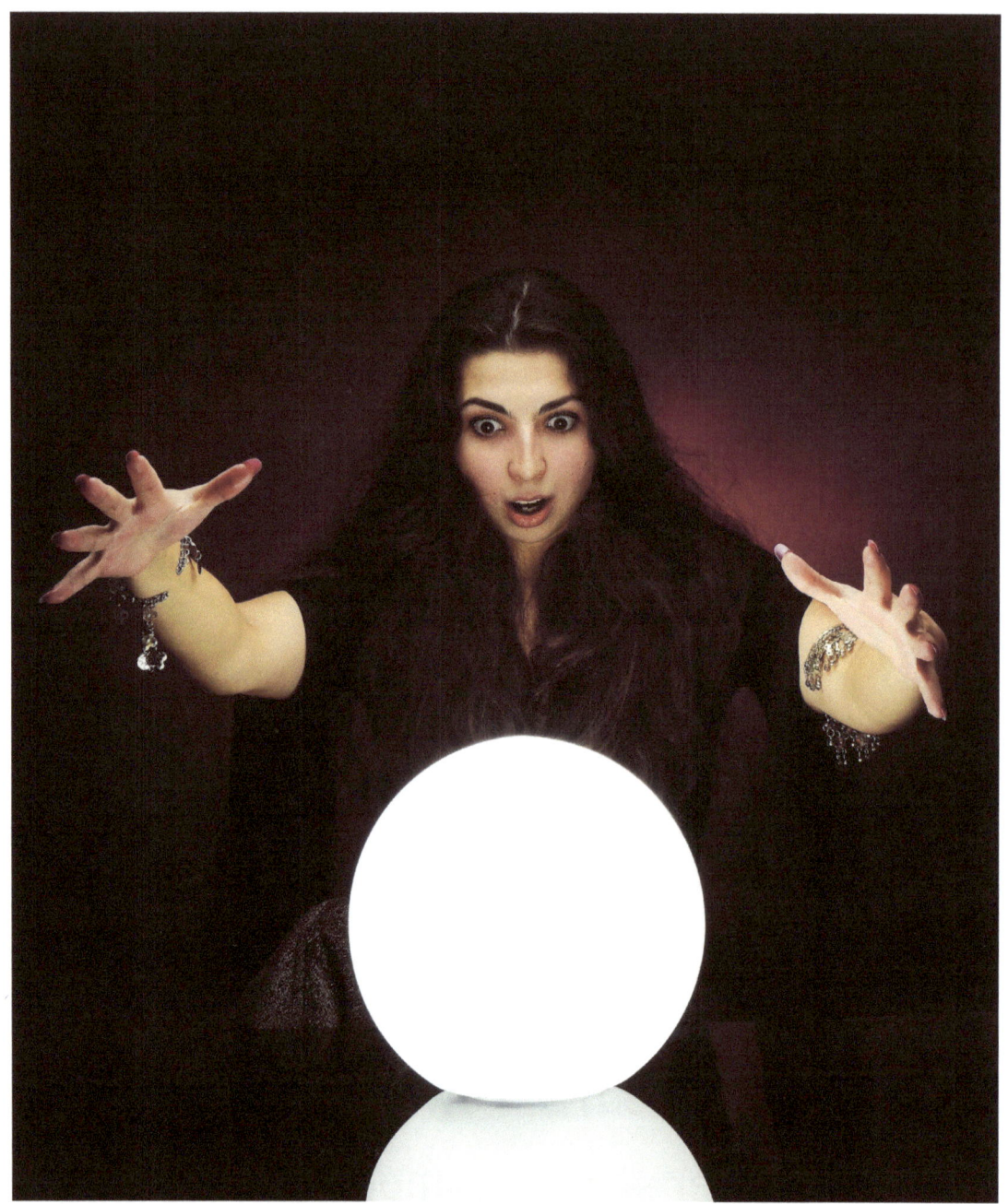

Before considering what Hypnosis is, perhaps it would be appropriate to establish what it................ is not

Hypnosis is *not "mind control."*

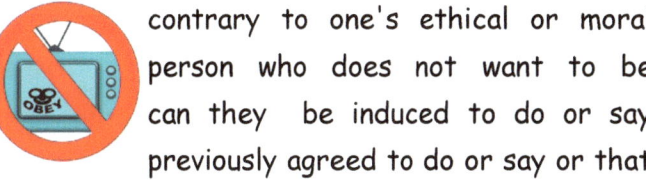

A Hypnotic suggestion that is contrary to one's ethical or moral standards is inherently ineffectual. A person who does not want to be Hypnotized cannot be Hypnotized nor can they be induced to do or say anything, which they have not previously agreed to do or say or that which violates their personal standards of behavior or integrity. There is neither magic nor coercion involved. Any Hypnotist can explain the actions or behaviors produced on stage for entertainment. Much of the subject matter seen in films or TV is simply fiction.

Hypnosis is *not miraculous*

It certainly will aid the therapeutic process if the client has "faith" in the practitioner and his ability to help them to make the changes they desire.

Hypnosis will enable *your client' to exploit their subconscious* mind's characteristics more productively.

Hypnosis does not weaken the will power. It can actually strengthen it.

Hypnosis *does not require sleep or a loss of consciousness* to be effective.

A Hypnosis subject may fall asleep during a Hypnotic session and still benefit. The subconscious mind never sleeps. In most cases the subject is fully aware of communication and is able to respond or request either verbally or by signal nor is unconsciousness involved. A subject, when asked to make a specific movement will comply with the request unless it is objectionable in which case there will be a refusal. The subject is in complete and total control of himself/herself while in the Hypnotic state.

No one can be permanently kept in the Hypnotic state against their will. When Hypnotic suggestion are no longer being administered, the subject will eventually emerge from Hypnosis naturally.

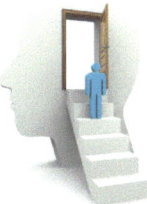

Everyone is capable of entering Hypnosis.

…..It is believed that a higher IQ facilitates certain Hypnotic procedures;Conversely it has been demonstrated that the lower, facilitates other beneficial outcomes

In actuality, all Hypnosis is Self Hypnosis. While in Hypnosis, subjects allow changes, based on the suggestions and information previously agreed to then projected by the Hypnotist into their subconscious. The objectives are determined 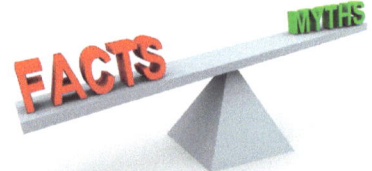 and agreed to during the preconditioning phase. Hypnosis is actually a "Mutual endeavor." The success of its objective will depend upon the cooperation and trust between the participants,as we will define in "Building Rapport"

The unconscious mind cannot differentiate between fact and fiction.

It relies on the conscious mind for that ability. Successful Hypnosis is accomplished with Positive Suggestions. Suggestions are directed to the unconscious, either passively *(indirect)* or very commandingly *(authoritarian)*, while the client is in a Hypnotic trance.

We are already influenced with many negative or undesirable suggestions on a day to day basis through television news the web and radio or from some the people we come in contact with.SO....

Hypnosis can provide Positive, Beneficial, Voluntary, replacement attitudes, suggestions and reflexes.

An actual Success story: (This program if further described in the Scripts section of this manual).

Back into the World !

The Client, a middle aged married woman with degrees in business and finance, 2 children in college, with a desire to resume a career, contacted me regarding Hypnosis as an aid to loose weight.

Her self described self image was so low as to influence all aspects of her daily personal and social and possible, business life.

She no longer felt attractive or even personable. Her energy level and attitude was such that she had difficulty in establishing any sort of physical activity or light exercise.

We scheduled a "Mutual Evaluation and Demonstration" appointment.

During this appointment we established her weight loss goals and that there were no obvious apparent medical consideration to losing 30 lbs.

If I have even the slightest doubt that there may be a reason to consider the advisability of a significant weight loss I insist upon the written approval of a Medical professional.

The first session was approximately 45 minutes long, and was primary to determine her actual willingness to enter into a state of Hypnosis.

We were very successful. I gave her some positive relaxing suggestions.

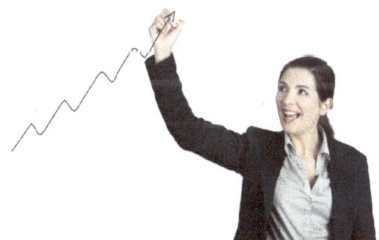

The result of this Interview and successful induction was her commitment to a 30 day weight loss series, commencing on the second day, with Hypnosis sessions every other day for a total of 15 sessions while implementing other proprietary aspects of a lifetime weight loss and maintenance program offered here at the Florida Holistics Institute.

Three months Later, as a result of attaining her weight loss goal and its maintenance, she called and enrolled in another series designed to enhance her public speaking effectiveness.... *Back into the World!!*

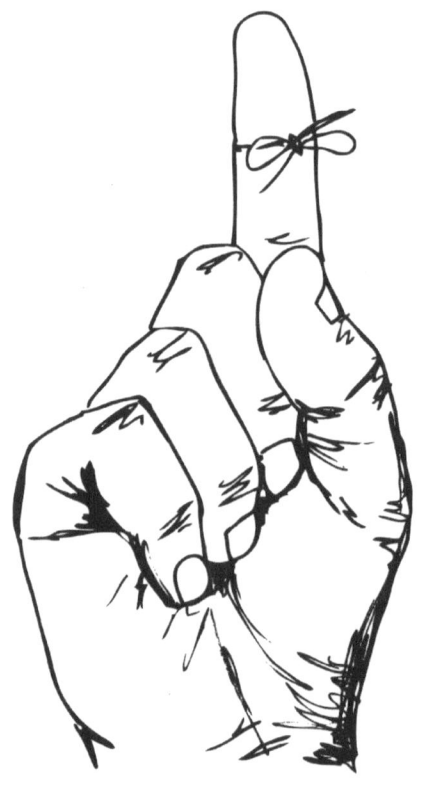

Understanding Memory

Memory is the storage and retrieval of previous experience, or the ability to recall our thoughts. We now understand that the size of the human mind is such that it could not be filled in a total lifetime.

Stored memories last a lifetime

3 Categories of memory

Today's science has determined that Memory storage involves at least three distinct categories; short- term (**STM**) memory and long term (**LTM**) memory and Sensory Memory **(SEM)**. Short term memory is a fleeting memory, lasting for seconds to a few hours. It is the preliminary step to long term memory. *The primary function of sleep is thought to be the consolidation of information.* This concept is utilized in a PBHI proprietary technique taught in this course.

STM can be illustrated by remembering a telephone number for a few seconds, usually limited to 7 or 8 separate bits but then it cannot be recalled. Short-term memory is supported by transient patterns of neuronal communication, dependent on regions of the frontal lobe (especially dorsolateral prefrontal cortex) and the parietal lobe.

The **STM** unaided, can not recall a number much longer than that of a phone number. We can remember significant phone numbers by consciously making an effort to committing them to long-term memory. Long-term memories, on the other hand, are maintained by more stable and permanent changes in neural connections widely spread throughout the brain. The <u>hippocampus</u> is considered essential to the consolidation of information from short-term to long-term memory. Although it does not seem to store information itself, the hippocampus has been found to be involved in changing neural connections for a period of three months or more after the initial learning

........*In contrast to **STM**, long-term memory (**LTM**) which seems to have an unlimited capacity and to date, an undefined structure.*

*Sensory Memory **(SEM)** holds sensory information for a few seconds or less after an item is perceived. The ability to look at an item, and remember what it looked like with just a second of observation, or memorization, is an example of sensory memory. It is out of cognitive control and is an automatic response*

To prevent overload, our conscious mind decides what information is important and what is not.

Episodically reinforced memories **(ERM)** are automatically sent to long-term storage. An example of this would be the 911 attack. We remember where we were and what we were doing on that day. This is an episodically reinforced memory. We *can exploit this process In the Hypnotic state of heightened suggestibility (episodic).*

A long time ago, a phone number was given to me by a very attractive member of the opposite sex. It may never be forgotten. It was stored in my important file.

Long-and some short term memories, can be accessed in the Hypnotic state, reportedly, as far back as the birthing experience. *1
Even while we are sleeping or under anesthesia our unconscious mind is still recording events that can be accessed by the Hypnotic state.

Our ability to recall certain detailed information seems to improve with aging.

Summary

Hypnosis has the potential to change lives, by stimulating the learning process, increasing motivation, establishing beneficial study habits, boosting confidence, reducing study and test anxiety and accessing memory.

Hypnosis dealing with our modern understanding of memory can be a valuable tool for goal setting and achievement.

Altering the subconscious programming through positive suggestion in the susceptible state, Hypnosis subjects can change unwanted habits or addictions, enhance various attributes and relieve or manage pain.

All Hypnosis is SELF Hypnosis. The Hypnotist is merely a facilitator

Chapter One
Review questions

01......Hypnosis is Sleep..T..........F

02......All Hypnosis is self Hypnosis..T..........F

03......Dr. Braid Developed the basis for contemporary

Hypnosis..T..........F

04......LTM is the acronym for Long Term Motivation.................T..........F

05......Hypnosis is the relaxation of the conscious mind............T..........F

06......Sensory Memory is considered a conscious response......T..........F

07......Under Hypnosis, the subconscious mind will accept either
true or false information..T..........F

08......List here, the three Categories of Memory:.......

Briefly comment here regarding your answer to
Question # 7:...

Chapter 2

THE THEORETICAL DEPTH LEVELS OF HYPNOSIS

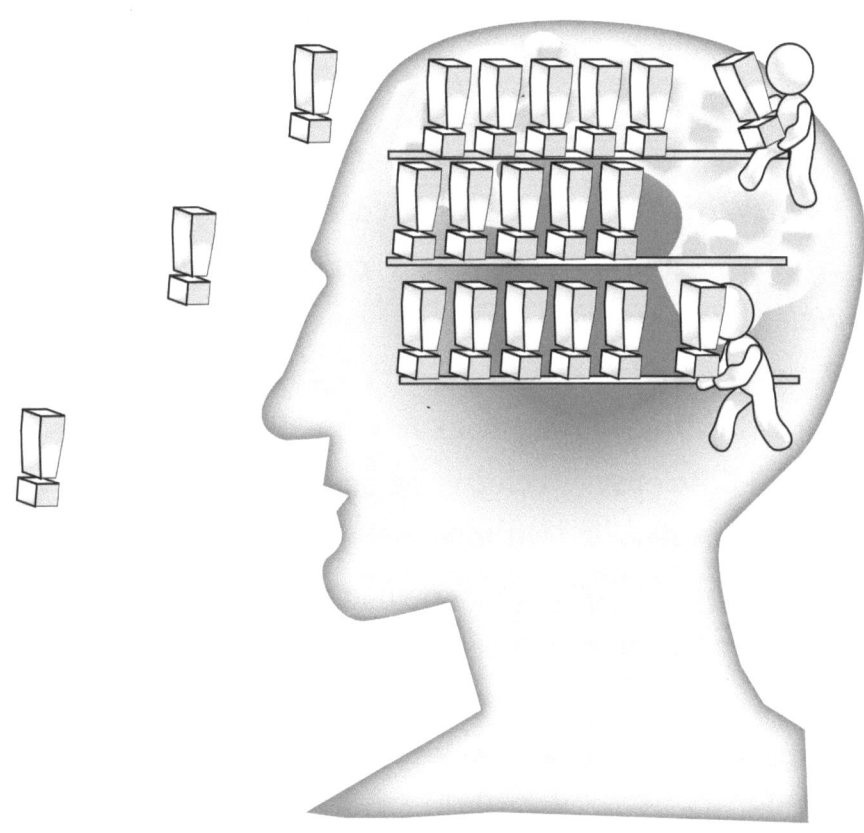

There are as many methods of judging trance levels as there are experimenters in Hypnosis.

Aron's Depth Scale (6 levels)

At one time only **three** levels were considered important which were Light, Medium and Deep.

Arron and others agreed that more specific and determinable degrees of differentiation are needed to identify the necessary levels at which to comfortably accomplish dental work, surgery, child-birthing and even age regression.

There are two Divisions of Aron's depth scale. Both contain three levels:
First: With three levels which are called *Mnemonic*-memory retaining.
*Second: **With three*** levels called, Amnesic – Described as Temporary Selective Amnesia.

A total of SIX <u>ARRON'S</u> LEVELS OF Hypnosis Level 1-1 Hypnoidal – So light that the subject does not feel Hypnotized, and feel awake but with Eyelid Catalepsy. Much can be accomplished even in this 1st level: weight reduction, smoking withdrawal, etc.

    Level 1-2 More relaxed, light relaxation. Larger muscle groups can be manipulated such as Arm Catalepsy. The beginning of critical reasoning impairment.

    Level 1-3 Fairly complete control of the entire muscular system can be established. Partial Analgesia can be induced. The subject can be convinced that they cannot rise from a chair, cannot walk, or that they are unable to articulate or remember a number, or upon awakening, Most Stage Hypnotists will not work with a subject unless they are in at least Level Three.

The first three levels are which most Clinical Hypnotists work with

Level 2-1 Beginning of Amnesic stages. A more profound level of the suggestibility phenomena is exhibited.

Level 2.2 Beginning of Somnambulism. Complete anesthesia is present The subject will feel neither pain nor touch. Positive hallucinations can be induced.

Level 2.3 Profound Hypnotic

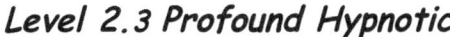

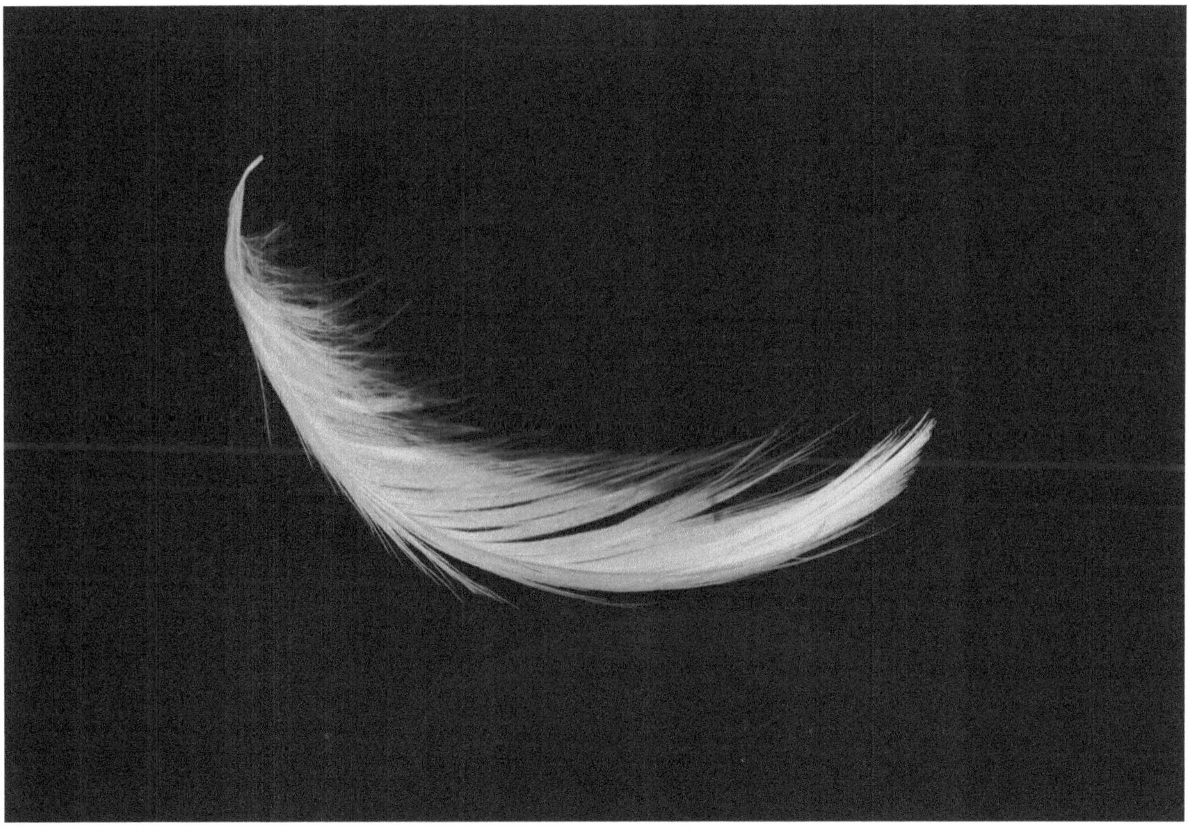

***Somnambulism.**[1]* *Characteristically the deepest state of Hypnosis. (Commonly referred to as level 6)*

*1 SOMNAMBULISM

Somnambulism is a <u>very</u> deep state of Hypnosis. A level 5 or 6 The persons at this level will seem asleep, Their breathing is noticeably slower. They exhibit great difficulty in enunciating words and If they are able to answer, they take a long time to answer, usually with a whisper. The subject, if asked would be unable to raise an arm or leg

In this state they have very limited recall of events during Hypnosis. Because of this, it is essential that you tell your client that " you should remember everything" It is possible that this person may be the 1 out of a 100 who is a somnambulistic. In this state they feel no pain at all, it is naturally and completely blocked. I personally have only witnessed 2 subjects in this state, One was the National Board directors wife who is a somnambulistic and worked at the board. They engaged in extensive research for years on this unusual state. The second was a no smoking client in my own clinic..

It is believed by some that 10 out of 100 women and that 10 out of 1,000 men are able to achieve this deep a level. We believe this is where the concept that Hypnosis is sleep originated, as at this level, the subjects do seem to be asleep. They are **NOT** asleep.

A person in this level will take suggestions much more readily and act on them for longer periods of time.

LEVEL TESTING

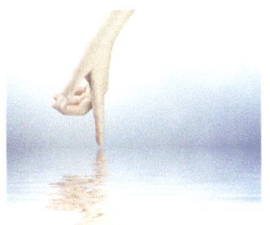

Depth stages are necessary in order to determine the level of analgesia or anesthesia necessary for dental work, surgery, child-birthing or for age regression.

. The lighter levels are all that are needed to accomplish behavior changes or in conjunction with psychotherapy.

In level testing, do not proceed to another *"challenge"* if previous *"challenges fail"*. Accept the level of the subject's aptitude for Hypnosis at this time and proceed, keeping in mind that each session will further deepen their trance depth

Suggested Lower Level Tests:

Eye Catalepsy The subject is told that they *Cannot open their eyes*

Arm Catalepsy The subject is told that they *Cannot lift an arm*

Number Block The subject is told that when counting from one to ten that they cannot remember any number after 5

Suggested Higher Level Tests:

Glove analgesia The subject is told that they will not feel pain, but will feel touch.

Most dental work, minor surgery. Can be performed, telling the subject that they will still feel air rushing into incision, slight pressure but no pain.

Positive hallucinations The subject is told to *see a clock on the wall with a fictitious time displayed*

Negative hallucinations The subject is told that they cannot to *see an object.*

Trance Levels:

Catalepsy: - *Muscular rigidity* can be experienced in first 3 stages in varying degrees.

Amnesia: - Divides the 3rd / 4th levels. 3therd level is the inability to articulate a number. at the 4th level most subjects can be told to forget a number.

Anesthesia - Divides the 4th and 5th levels: 4th level - analgesia - no pain but the sensation of pressure will be present

Complete anesthesia - 5th level neither pain nor pressure.

Hallucinations-
Positive hallucinations, seeing or hearing that which is not there.

Negative hallucinations- 6th level, not seeing or hearing specified objects or sounds.

5 Stages of a Hypnotherapy session

1. The pre-talk

"Rapport "[1] is established... A trusting relationship with the client. After the forms are filled out, engage in 15-30 minutes of evaluation time, determining suggestibility, observing the subject's personality and establishing the specific goals of the therapy session(s). Discuss finances at this point.

It is very important during your consultation that you listen carefully to and take note of and possibly record the subject's reasons for consulting you, their speech patterns, physical posture, grooming, dress style and heed any subliminal signals you may feel to produce empathy and establish a comfortable communication environment with the client.

2. Induction

Use a prepared Progressive Relaxation, Induction script or procedure and optionally, Guided Imagery, audio stimulus, with subliminal augmentation to induce the subject into the Hypnotic trance.

3. Deepening

A procedure used to encourage the client to relax into a deeper level of trance. A common deepening is counting.

4. Suggestion

The operative segment of a Hypnosis session, where directives for positive change are made from Predetermined Suggestions with Anchoring Techniques and Triggers.

5. Awakening

Gradually directing the subject out of Hypnosis. A Post-Talk segment should be included at this time.

RAPPORT

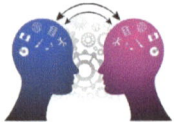

Rapport is the process of reflecting the client's behavior in such a way that trust is created. It is done with matching and mirroring behavior, as well as by empathy and understanding.

Under Hypnosis, the subject will experience a state of restricted attention to some or all stimuli residing in their normal field of awareness. Rapport, enhances this hyper suggestibility and the operator's suggestions are followed more readily but proportional to the client's belief and confidence established by the operator. This is a special kind of relationship, and must be conducted carefully and responsibly as the attention paid to the words of the operator, result in the subject usually responding with pinpoint literalness or specificity especially if they are in accord with his wishes and needs.

Whenever this *state of communication* is established between the operator and a subject, a suggestion or information will be accepted.

Some subjects in good rapport will even respond to an operator's Hypnotically installed suggestions in a printed or written format.

Blind people and deaf mutes can be Hypnotized through other sensory modalities if there is good rapport.-

Most subjects after experiencing stage 4 will respond to the voice of the operator over the telephone, or in a text message provided they have been conditioned for this posthypnotic response. Some therapists have used an associate without prior training in Hypnotic techniques, to produce, in a preconditioned client, upon a prearranged trigger, deep Hypnosis in a willing subject.

It has been said that the rapport in Hypnosis is due to emotional dependency on the operator. There is no more dependency in the Hypnotic-situation than in any other psycho therapeutic relationship. When auto (or self) Hypnosis is incorporated into therapy, whatever dependency exists is minimized or eliminated.

The success of all Hypnotherapy is based on a good interpersonal relationship. It is essential that Both the operator and patient enter into good rapport, since it provides each with emotional satisfaction that otherwise could not be obtained. More research should be directed toward the most essential psychological phenomena of Hypnosis-- Rapport.

One can conclude from the above that the patient's rapport denotes the ability and willingness of the patient to enter into an intensified communication with the operator. As a result, the subject is conditioned to accept the confidence that is so necessary for the establishment of Hypnotic induction, exploiting the Hypnotic state to instill beneficial behavioral responses and changes.-

Extend careful attention to this phase of every session.

The American Medical Association has reported that 40% to 60% of all "*cures*" are the result of the rapport between patients and doctors.

IE: *"The Placebo Effect", Is a Mal-named description of the phenomenon in which,, 40 to 50 percent of a medication's effect is not attributable to the medication.*

1994, Irving Kirsch distinguished Hypnosis as a *"non deceptive placebo," i. e., a method that openly makes use of suggestion and employs methods to amplify its effects* Kirsch, I. (1994). "Clinical Hypnosis as a non deceptive placebo: Empirically derived techniques". *The American journal of clinical Hypnosis*

MODELING, MIRRORING AND PACING

There are several ways that you can build rapport with your client. The most common are Modeling, Mirroring and Pacing,.often taught in NLP**1 classes however their existence precedes NLP by many years.

Modeling

Modeling is probably the most popular and traditional method of working with others. It is simply taking the position you would like the other person to match, speaking to them in the *manner* and *tense* you wish them to respond.

The Modeler may be enthusiastic while the Modeled is depressed, or calm while the subject is excited, Resolute, while the client is indecisive.

Mirroring

Mirroring is the technique you employ when you want to show a person that you are sympathetic, and not threatening. A subtle mirroring of another's body movements will imply sympathy. People in agreement unconsciously assume the same posture, using similar gestures and tempo.

If your client is agitated, depressed, defensive, or tense, Initially, very subtly assume the same position and mannerisms, then as you establish the beginning of rapport again, subtly change your posture and your mannerisms to create a more positive position. Your clients will unconsciously change their postures and mannerisms to match yours.

Verbal Mirroring

Verbal mirroring is more complex. You can be quite effective if you concentrate on the tone and tempo of your client's voice. When you can match it, the results are quite profound.

**1=Neural- Linguistic Programming

PACING

Pacing, to quote Dr. Milton Erickson,* means *"meeting people where they are by reflecting what they know or assume to be true or by matching some part of their ongoing experience."* Pacing is used in concert with modeling and mirroring, and, more simply put, allows you to voluntarily enter your client's world for a brief moment for the purpose of leading him toward his stated goal. One way to do this is to ask questions that can only be answered, "*Yes*" or whatever other response you desire.

An example of this would be as follows: If you to a new car dealership to look at new cars and the salesman said to you "nice day today is it not?" Yes. "Your baby is very pretty isn't she?" Yes. He continued until you agree multiple times and then he would say:

"if I could get this car for you at a monthly payment would you take it today ?"

Subliminal Messaging Under Hypnosis

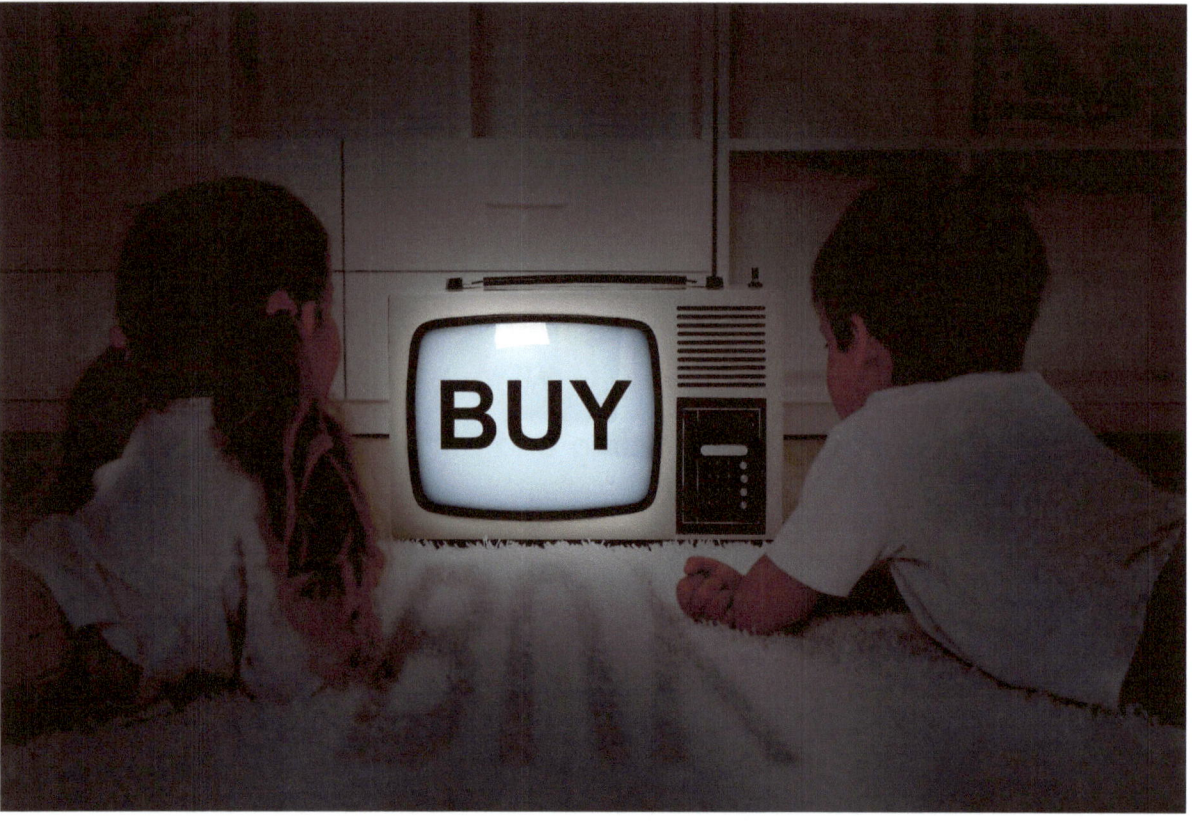

Dr. Lloyd H. Silverman, a psychologist at New York University, has been at the forefront of subliminal testing for over 20 years Has found that a group exposed to subliminal messages had a <u>five times greater chance of quitting smoking</u> than the group not exposed to subliminal messages.
One month after the study 66% percent group exposed to subliminal messages were still non-smokers, compared to 13% of the control group.
It is important *that the Hypnotist first check local jurisdictions and obtain a signed client's consent statement before initiating any subliminal actions.*
PBHI *has developed subliminal techniques using The SHARM audio software described in the Office/Clinic section of this manual and provides in-clinic instruction with recommended software and hardware to fully exploit Video and Audio Subliminals to used during in Clinic sessions.*

THE RECOGNITION AND CLASSIFICATION OF SUBJECTS

Every normal person is able to be Hypnotized. Roughly 15 percent of the population is held to be highly resistant. The operative word is *Normal.*

Exceptions:
Infants and children under age 3 or 4.......do not have a sufficient attention span.

Psychotics- Generally not good subjects, and if under medication there seems to be limited attention span and little documented benefit from Hypnosis.

Mentally retarded - with an IQ under 70
beneficial Hypnosis Can be accomplished in a clinical environment.

Paranoiaclly inclined, It is Possible in a clinical setting, to Hypnotize distrustful, suspicious personalities with beneficial results. (It is suspected that habitual cannabis usage will induce or exacerbate a paranoid personality.) In such situations, a trance state will be very difficult to achieve.

People over 80......some, are more difficult to work with but the results of relieving anxieties are very rewarding personally for the Hypnotherapist.

Common Popular Misconceptions

Strong willed Hypnotist - weak willed subject.
FALSE!

Regardless of what the client wants, they will be Hypnotized.
FALSE!

A person in Hypnosis **will do anything you tell them**………
FALSE!

A person in Hypnosis **always tells the truth**………………
FALSE

Control---A Hypnotist does not control the subject. Explain to your clients that the Hypnotist is only a guide.
The power is supplied by the client.

A person in Hypnosis can safely perform exceptional demonstrations of strength………………………….False

SUSCEPTIBILITY

One of the most widely used scales was described in 1959 by Stanford's Hilgard.

In the Stanford Hypnotic Susceptibility Scales, subjects who undergo Hypnotic induction are given 12 suggestions--imagine a mosquito buzzing around, imagine a weight in one hand--while the Hypnotist watches for evidence of responsiveness such as shifting position to avoid the insect. On a scale of zero (not hypnotizable) to 12 (highly so), subjects are scored by the degree of their response to the 12 suggestions

A Monotonous environment is conducive. Monotonous tasks can keep the level of concentration in one channel, *IE*: assembly line workers.

Women are more open to Hypnosis.

People out of their own environment such as when in a doctor's office tend to develop a respectful, expectant, attitude. A professional office setting is a facilitating environment.

Once a person agrees to accept the role of a Hypnotic subject, the outcome is highly predictable. Some subjects get so deeply involved that they feel as though they no longer have a choice in the matter. The Client's acceptance of their role as a Hypnotic subject possibly involves a willing suspension of some of their own preconceptions.

PERSONALITY CONSIDERATIONS

A Sensitive, neurotic, tense person who can't concentrate, has trouble sleeping, temperamental, can't relax.

A Calm, relaxed, controlled, person who sleeps well, normal, set in his ways and is apparently quite stable emotionally

Which one is more susceptible to Hypnosis?

Neither characteristic is a valid description of a more susceptible Personality

Limiting Disrupting Factors

Physical discomfort of any kind is a hindrance.

Apprehension Be aware of the signs such as Perspiration or cold, clammy skin. Review and increase your rapport effort.

Coughing will interrupt a trance.

Physical exhaustion tends to increase the tendency for the subject to go into natural sleep.

.. **Intoxication** or Prescribed Medication is definitely unfavorable The influence of prescribed or street drugs will obstruct or divert the Hypnotheraputic Effort..
(Drugs are legitimately used in some Professional Medical Clinical environments).This is a very controversial matter

Certain **types of fear** of th e operator such as fascination or awe. can be a favorable influence,

AGE Considerations

4 - 10 is the most suggestible age – but difficult unless you understand and specialize in children.

18 - 21 is a period of uneven emotional growth among most potential subjects the ability to be Hypnotized readily, varies

Subjects 21 and up potentially, will realize the most recognizable benefits from Hypnosis.

There is a gradual decline in susceptibility with advanced age

All age groups have been found to be very receptive to Hypnotic relaxation suggestions and pain management."

De Pascalis, V.; Magurano, M.R.; Bellusci, A. (1999)." somatosensory perception, event-related potentials and skin conductance to painful stimuli in high, mid, and hypnotizable subjects: Effects of differential pain Pain strategies

SUGGESTIBILITY TESTING

Suggestibility tests are not as useful in a professional setting as an *extensive rapport effort,* which is more effective and will also provide clues from the subject's responses for the most suitable Hypnotic induction method to use.

Chevreul's Pendulum

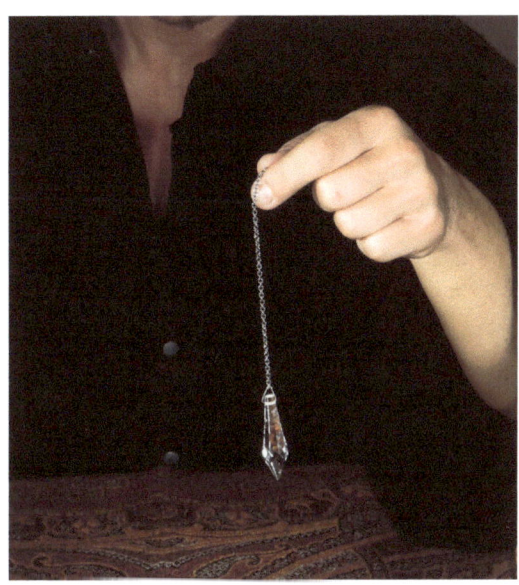

A test of Concentration (a permissive test).
This test is named after an early French Hypnotist. It is an excellent initial test because it is successful with most clients. It is an especially good test for children.

Significance of Subject's Response:

Positive response – The pendulum will move exactly in the suggested direction

Negative response-No movement or movement contrary to the suggestion, indicating a resistance. Hypnosis is contraindicated.

The Falling Backward 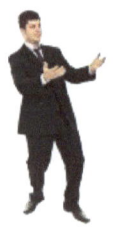 Test

This test is very authoritative and is primarily used by Stage Hypnotists. As it requires touching

*Your tone should be very authoritative as this is a test of **Trust**.*

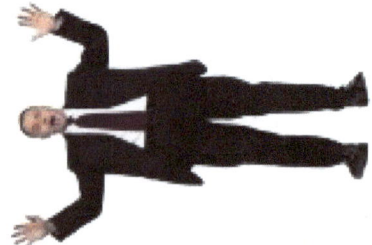

Negative Outcome sound = *A dull Thud* ;-)

Group Demonstrations

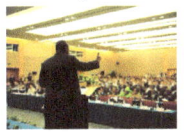

The Arms Rising and Falling Test

This is a very effective preconditioning aid, demonstrating Hypnotic suggestibility. Imagination is the most potent force in Hypnosis.

You have a good imagination, don't you? Good! Then I'd like to do a process to see how well you can use your imagination.

If you would, please stand up. Could you step back just a bit? Good, Thank you. Let your arms hang loosely at your side. That's it. Just relax now and let your arms hang loosely at your side.

Now, I'd like you to please close your eyes. If you will, raise your arms forward and upward to shoulder level. Good! Please turn your left hand up so that your left palm faces the ceiling. Now, extend your right thumb up so that your right thumb points up at the ceiling. Good!

This is a process in **imagination**, so what I would like you to do now is *imagine* In your mind's eye or even pretend if you have to, that: In your left palm you have a very heavy book.

At the same time, *imagine* attached to your right thumb is a string. The string is attached to a large, red helium balloon. Helium is a gas that rises, it will cause your right hand to go up, up, up, up; while the heavy book takes your left hand down, down, down, Right hand going up, up, up, up, and left hand going down, down, down. Right hand going up, up, up, up. Left hand going down, down, down, down, right hand going up, up, up, up.

Now, please open your eyes. Did you notice that your left hand went down, and your right hand went up? If it did, this test would indicate that you have a good imagination.

Significance of this Group's Responses:

Positive response – Most participants arms move in a slow and deliberate manner, Indicating a successful Hypnotic influence.

Negative response - rapid movement of arms in an upward or downward direction would indicate the subjects trying to please the Hypnotist.

No movement - would indicate extreme resistance.

Rarely, You may observe a subject's hands moving in the opposite direction suggested, some psychologists consider this an indication of a form of Dyslexia.

Hand Clasp Test

This test could be applied if you find your client not responding well with the permissive tests. It is also an excellent method to use when demonstrating suggestibility testing with groups. At the beginning of this test, ask your clients take off any rings that may interfere. At the conclusion, ask for feedback from your client.- Start this test in a normal speaking voice and change the tone to a more forceful authoritative manner......

An authoritative test of imagination

*Please put everything down, and sit facing me. Extend your **clasped** hands in front of you with your elbows locked.*

Push your hands forward, just as though you're pushing through the wall in front of you. Focus your attention on your crossed thumbs. Now, I'd *like you to **imagine** your hands are in a vise, and the vise is closing and tightening. **Imagine** that your hands are fusing together, stuck like glue. Stuck tighter and tighter together, tighter and tighter your knuckles are getting whiter and whiter, as your hands press closer and closer. Tighter and tighter together, whiter and whiter, your hands are now stuck together like glue. Stuck so tightly together that in a moment I'm going to ask you to try to pull them apart and you'll find that you cannot. They'll be so tightly stuck together that you will be unable to pull them apart.*

*I'm going to count to three and at the count of three you'll try to pull them apart, and you'll find you **cannot**. Your hands are stuck tightly together, **stuck** like glue.*

<u>One</u> *- Tighter and Tighter*

<u>Two</u> *- Stuck together like glue.*

<u>Three</u> *- Try to pull them apart - You Cannot! Try! You Cannot!*

Now stop trying, relax and allow your hands to come apart.

Caution!-During a Hypnosis Session

Problems can occur which are similar to that encountered by doctors, dentists, psychologists, and psychiatrists. There is the possibility of being sued by a Litigious individual claiming that something illegal immoral or of a sexual nature occurred.

Intelligently observe professional procedures and standards and acquire malpractice insurance.

It is very important to realize Hypnosis can be erotic. Arousal of emotions under Hypnosis can occur, and can cause possible distracting, compromising, situations.

To avoid the above problems, it is a good idea to always have a signed tape / video recording agreement and the equipment in view. Answer possible client objection to recording by stating it may be necessary for reviewing the session at a later time. Indicate again on the intake form that you reserve the right to record the sessions.

If a more serious problem is suspected, it might be necessary to have someone else present, or at least be within earshot. If any sort of sexual arousal or distress is encountered, it is important to keep soothing dialog going. Say *"remain calm, peaceful, relaxed, and tranquil"*. Do not continue to use words suggesting Hypnosis. Do not continue any form of Hypnosis until calming has taken place. Always remember,

Do not bring the subject out until they are calm.

You can continue with the session. Or after calming, take them out and discontinue the use of Hypnosis.

If a client is not emerging from Hypnosis

Continue to give reassuring tones and commands, to bring them out. Speak louder and say, "I will have to charge another $xxx.00 if you don't come out of Hypnosis", However, Do not worry, the subject will eventually either come out of Hypnosis by themselves, or fall into natural sleep and then wake up normally.

Subliminal Suggestions

In 1974 the US **government banned subliminal advertising in commercials** because it was determined that influencing people without their knowledge was contrary to the public interest. The British, Australian, and Canadian Government have since followed suit. However,

When used for personal development, and with a signed consent form it is probably safe and legal. You must <u>first</u> check with your local authorities

Never induce full body catalepsy with weights placed on subjects.
Induce catalepsy gradually. This is very dangerous and could result in ruptures or permanent body injury. Physical stress or strain in waking state is exactly the same under Hypnosis and will be a source of danger in a Hypnotic state. Hypnosis does not give subjects strength (*physical*) that they do not possess. You can convince a person in Hypnosis that they are stronger and they could seriously damage themselves.

Age regression can bring on emotional outbursts. Age regression is a very valuable tool in short term therapy, to uncover repressed materials. It might be useful to inform a psychologist in your area of your availability to help them in this procedure.

In case of an emergency: <u>CALMLY</u> move to an awakening script.

Avoid sudden shocks Such as announcements of emotionally disturbing subjects or suggestions.

Never, *under Hypnosis* change subject's emotions suddenly which Some stage Hypnotists do for entertainment. Sudden induced emotional changes can seriously disturb an individual who may be in a sensitized state of mind.

Do not touch the client. Do not get out of your chair unless absolutely-necessary .

(The Legal Exceptions are Licensed Health care Professionals)

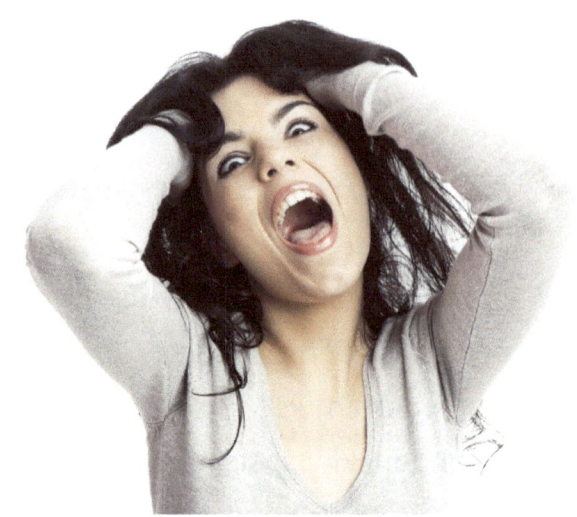

Unqualified Therapy is very dangerous

A Therapist Has special qualifications, specific licensure, training and in most jurisdictions is licensed in dealing with and managing emotional or mental health problems.

A Hypnotist: <u>only</u> trained in Hypnosis, <u>does not</u> qualify for handling emotional or mental health problems.

In Florida and Texas do not use the word **"*therapy*"**) unless licensed as a health care professional. It is important to work only within your realm of training, with guidelines set by your own qualifications.

A Real danger of unqualified therapy is that it may delay the use of necessary therapy or more serious damage

Chapter Two

Review questions

01.....Rapport is not essential to induce Hypnosis..T..........F

02.....The most effectively Hypnotized age group is 21 to 75 Years of age...T..........F

03.....NLP is Neural Linguistic Programming..T..........F

04.....Suggestibility tests are an essential element of
the pre-Hypnosis interview..T..........F

05.....Amnesia is experienced in the first level of Hypnosis......................T..........F

06.....Hypnosis and ESP are essentially the same.......................................T..........F

07.....Never raise your voice while the subject is under Hypnosis...........T..........F

08.....In Florida, as well as most other states you may treat with Hypnosis an emotionally induced skin rash without a physician's oversight............T..........F

09....Arron's depth scales were developed to define Insurance reimbursement rates..T..........F

10.....Somnambulism starts at depth level 3...T..........F

Ch 2 assignment:

Write:

Three original suggestions for a client who wants to lose weight

1

2

3

CHAPTER THREE

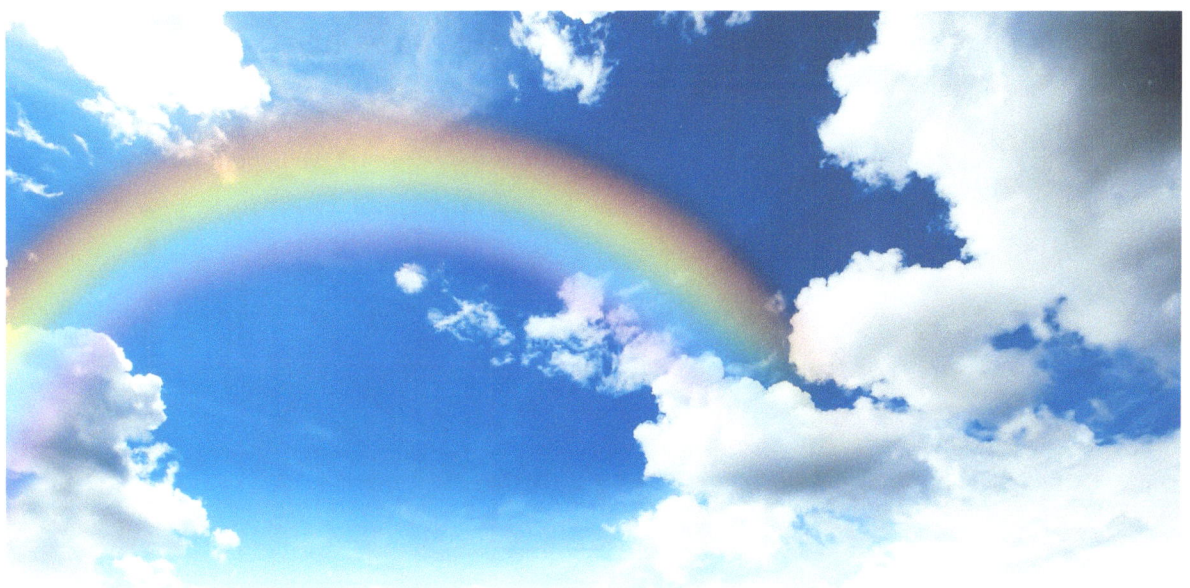

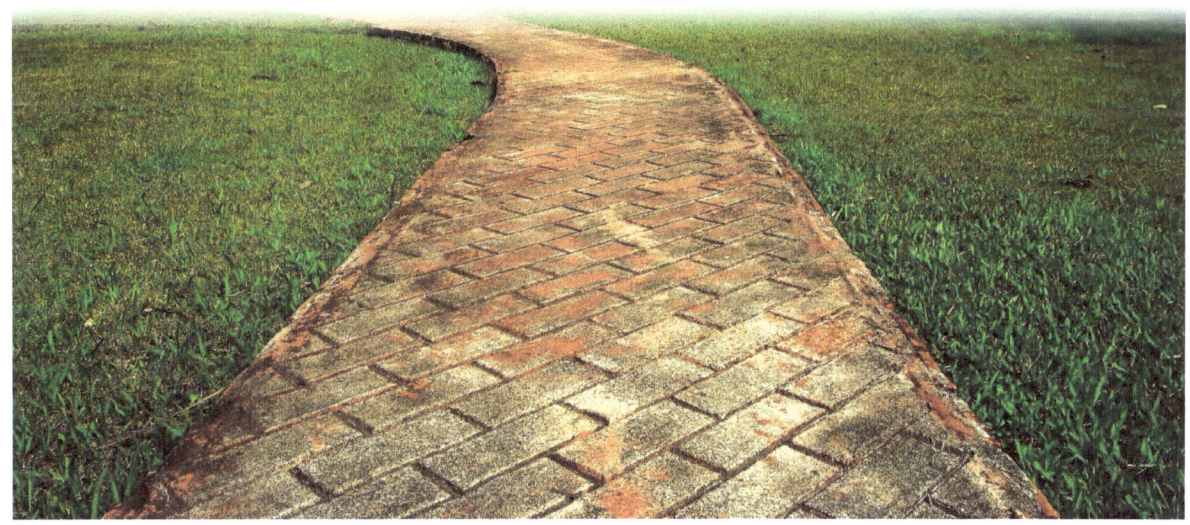

The Session.

Some Hypnosis sessions can last only fifteen minutes. Brief sessions are often used primarily by psychotherapists to induce clients to "open up" in a psychotherapy session or up to an hour or more for other objectives. Some types of regression therapy may last over two hours. But optimally, a standard session will last from 45 minutes to one hour.

Each Hypnotist will develop their own scripts resulting in reported rates of effectiveness varying from 40% to 95%. Today most Clinical practitioners prefer to use the progressive relaxation process to induce Hypnosis . As you develop your skills, you will develop your own specific style. This manual provides you with exposure to our wide range of proven techniques and resources to further your exploration of Hypnosis.

Factors to consider in a Hypnosis Session
A Hypnotist does not fail……. The subject may not consent.
Even a novice will achieve a 40% initial success rate and with experience, almost 100%
We do know that a person does not know when they are in Hypnosis. Hypnosis does not start or end anyplace! It is really the ability of a person to accept uncritically their own belief! It is a voluntary reaction more completely exercising their own ability.

A Hypnotist **must** exude **self-confidence** and professionalism……..create a positive environment, to create success…….Incremental insight is important. Refine your technique, language, rhythm and rapport.

Upon completion of this course and with practice, you will achieve 100% success.

Computer, Mechanical and Audio-Visual aids

Advanced technology and the expanded scientific understanding of the human brain and behavior, have greatly enhanced the effectiveness of Ethical Hypnosis.

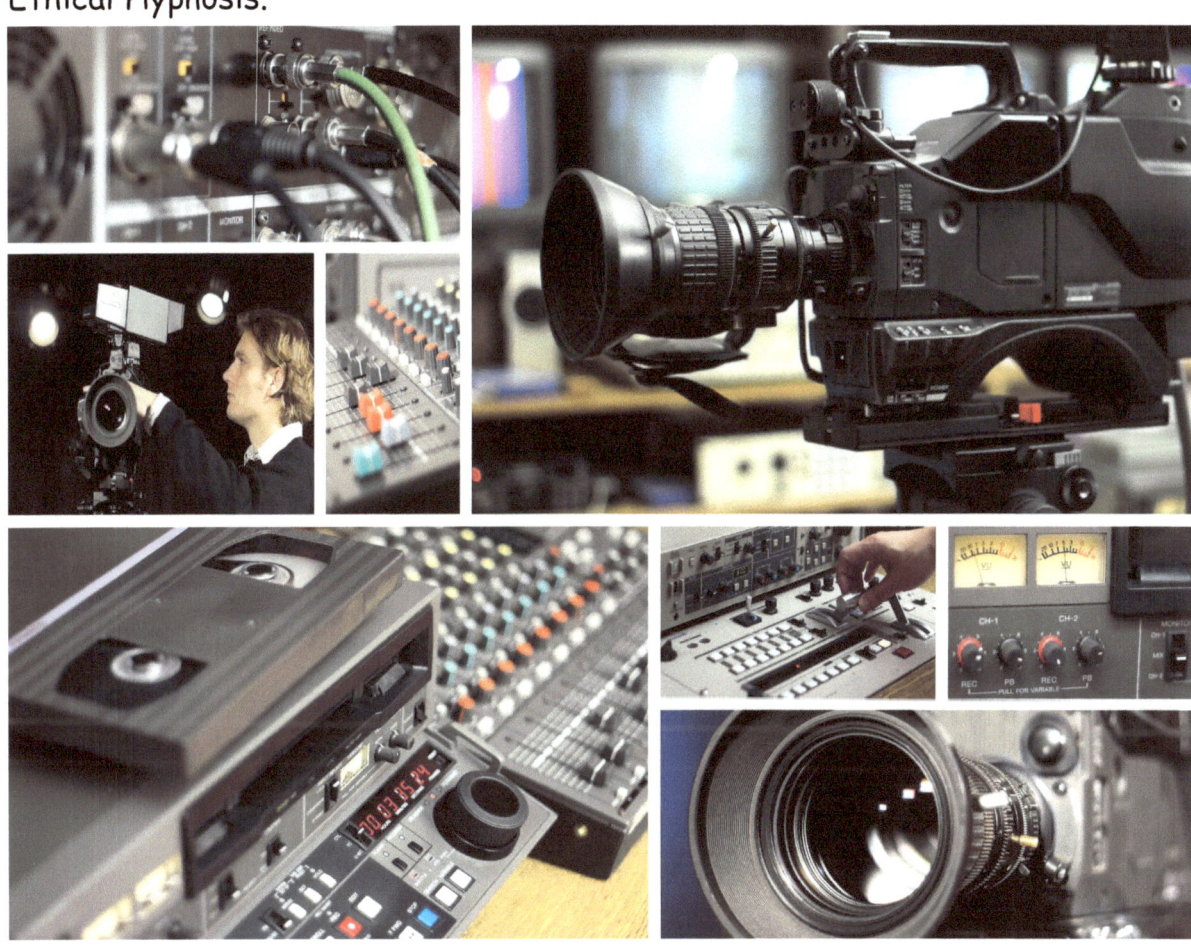

Professionally designed computer software applications for the Hypnotherapist will significantly augment the Therapist's modalities with selectable, scientifically authentic, multilevel, Hypnotic communication and metaphoric choices of sound and visual stimuli. to bring about rapid and lasting changes for your clients.

Versatile **Visual Trance** software is used during induction to present scientifically applied visual subliminal commands.
It is specifically designed to enable the Therapist to selectively modify, add or delete effects

Audio Enhancing and editing software with similar capabilities, is today, in a modern Clinical environment, essential.

At The Florida Holistics Institute our policy is to constantly evaluate and implement leading edge, state of the art, hardware, software and the results of responsible scientific, inquiry.
See.... Equipment, Software and environment list in chapter 5.

INDUCTIONS: *There has been a lot of progress in this field*

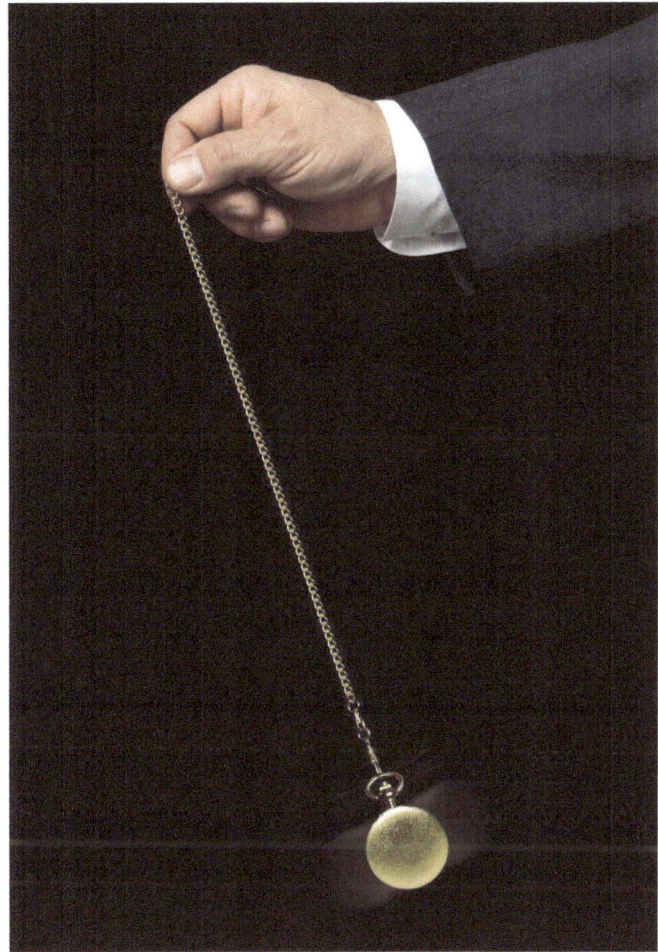

There are as many varieties of induction as there are Hypnotists.
This manual contains some proven methods. You should, with experience, personalize your methods within the framework described.
Also *See the recommended equipment list for state of the art equipment included in this manual*

Inductions

DR. FLOWER'S METHOD: Is a variation of the Repetition Principle; This is a very old and simple method. Please "Google" this method and others for your perspective.

The Eye Fixation Method: Say--"Look at the wall in front of you as though you are looking through the wall at a very pleasant scene.....look at the scene in a vague dreamy way". Using The Future Tense, Say "Soon you'll find all the muscle groups in your body will relax....your facial muscles will relax......your whole body will let go and soon you'll close your eyes and go into a sound, peaceful Hypnotic rest".

Then:-Take charge: take control.

"In a moment I'm going to count from one to twenty.....on each count, you'll close your eyes. In between counts you'll open your eyes. Some time before I reach the count of twenty, maybe at fifteen, maybe at nine, or perhaps three, you will be in a deep sound Hypnotic rest".

<u>Also Read:Master Secrets of Hypnosis</u> By Professor Kurt Tepperwein a 400+ page, comprehensive History of induction techniques The English version Library of congress catalog number is: 91 73801

A three Step Induction Procedure

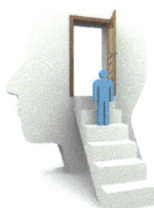

1. Preparatory Step: The Subject is told in **future tense** what to expect and what the impending signs of Hypnosis are: *You will become more and more relaxed. Your eyelids **will** become heavier, your eyes **will** become more tired, your breathing **will** become deeper and more regular."*

This is kept up anywhere from 1/2 minute to ten minutes, until the operator sees something happening, like: fixed stare, droopy eyes, sagging shoulders, body relaxed, etc. Then proceeds to the next step.

2. *Relaxation*

Switch to **Present Tense** - Extend the Assumption of Preparatory Step. Where the Hypnotist points out what he sees happening, and what should be happening:...."*Your eyes **are** starting to close. Your eyelids **are** heavier and heavier, you **are** more and more tired, more and more relaxed. You **are** becoming more and more relaxed, harder for you to keep your eyes open"* (this stage can also last from 1/2 minute to ten minutes, at which point the operator takes over).

3. *Take Charge:* Operator's voice becomes firmer, more emphatic. Takes over reins, establishes rapport, says forcefully, **now close your eyes and go down, deep, very deep into a Hypnotic rest!**" (Eyes may already be closed).

What should the subject be Experiencing ?

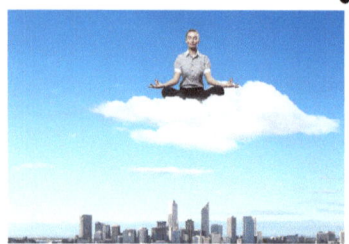

1. Effortless, directed Concentration: Little or no effort by the subject Concentration by itself is distracting! If a insomniac is told **"Go to Sleep"**, nothing would happen.
Verbiage for the Effortless Concentration stage could be:
" *Place your attention on the wall*" .

2. Fixation: In this stage the subject is literally hanging on every word said by the operator. "*Close your eyes and relax*".
If the operator were to leave the room, one of two things would happen; the subject would either emerge from Hypnosis or fall asleep. Hypnosis cannot be maintained without the operator/subject interaction. It has no persistence. The path into Hypnosis parallels the path into sleep.

3. The Passive State: Is that which can become the Hypnotic state as the Hypnotist establishes rapport.

> **4. Realization:** Under Hypnosis, when a subject realizes he cannot open his eyes for instance, this reinforces the belief in Hypnosis and tends to "*deepen the trance*".

Example: The subject is told, "*Try to open your eyelids, you cannot!*" and "*You will go deeper*". "*Try to raise your arm,--. You cannot!*" and Now, " *you will go deeper and deeper into Hypnosis*".

CONVINCERS

Hypnotist to Hypnotized Client.............

"*As you continue to relax, I am going to count from one to three. At the count of three you will find that you can't open your eyes, even if you try. You simply cannot open them. One, two, three. (the client tries to open their eyes.) That's fine. Don't even try anymore. Your doing so well now as you go deeper and deeper........*"

On three, look for a slight muscular pull in the client's eyelids. As soon as you see the effort, continue.

"*And as you go deeper, just concentrate on your left arm......Notice how heavy it is.....so heavy, very heavy. In fact, it is so heavy that when you try to lift it, it won't go up....just too heavy. (Client tries to lift arm) That's okay. It's just too much work.....don't even try anymore as you relax even more.......*"

Look for the effort. This is easy to spot by watching the arm for movement

The use of convincers is quite useful. When you are certain that the client is Hypnotized, it is recommended that you conduct a simple demonstration called

"*a convincer*" for the purpose of convincing the client, after the session, that they were indeed Hypnotized.

DEEPENING

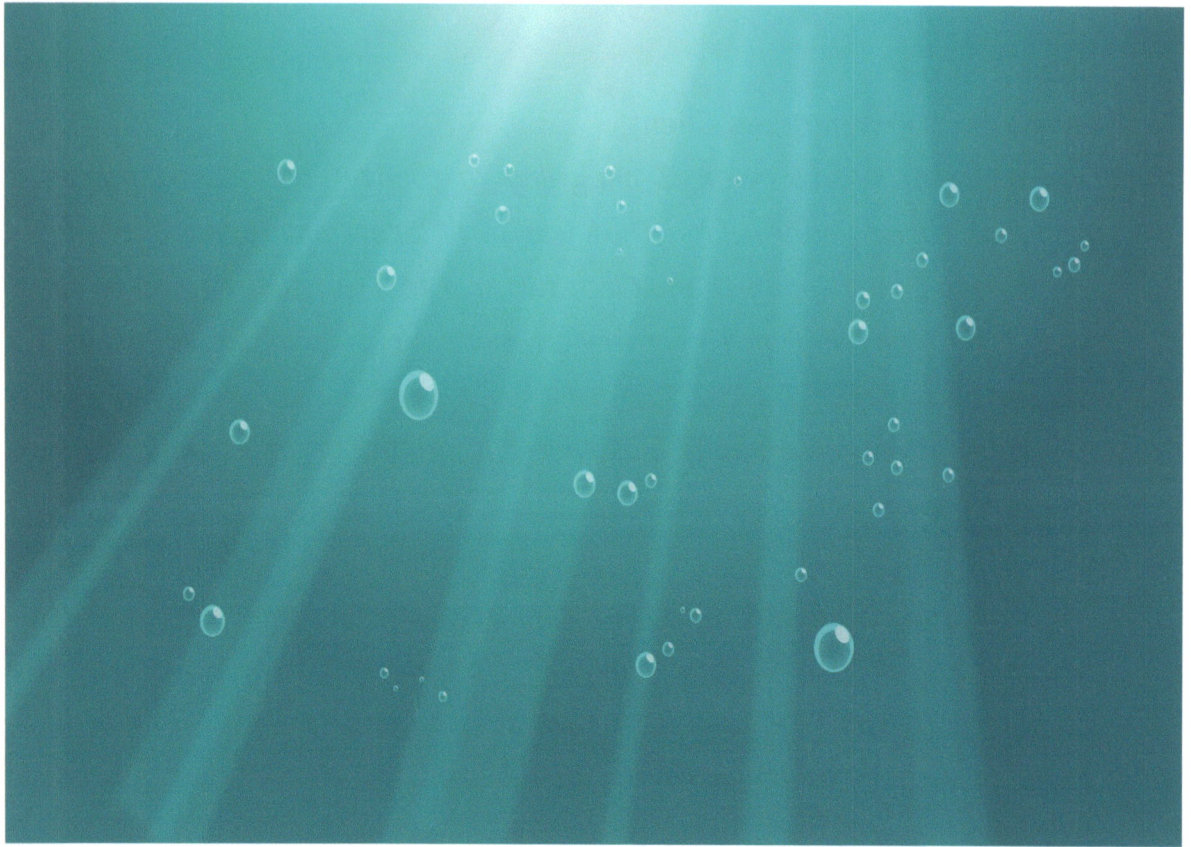

The Practice of Deepening is a ……………..controversial subject.

Many experienced Hypnotherapists will maintain that it can be more accurately described as a positive re-affirmation of the subject's actual presence in the Hypnotic state and that there is no real measurable "depth"

Repeated Deepening procedures Inductions are sometimes necessary to overcome some client's reservations....similar to the practice of various convincers..

see pg.72

The Whiteboard for Induction Intensification
To be used in most sessions For Critically analytical subjects, or people, with short attention spans **and** on every first session

(The Whiteboard) ***is a "Visualization Induction"***

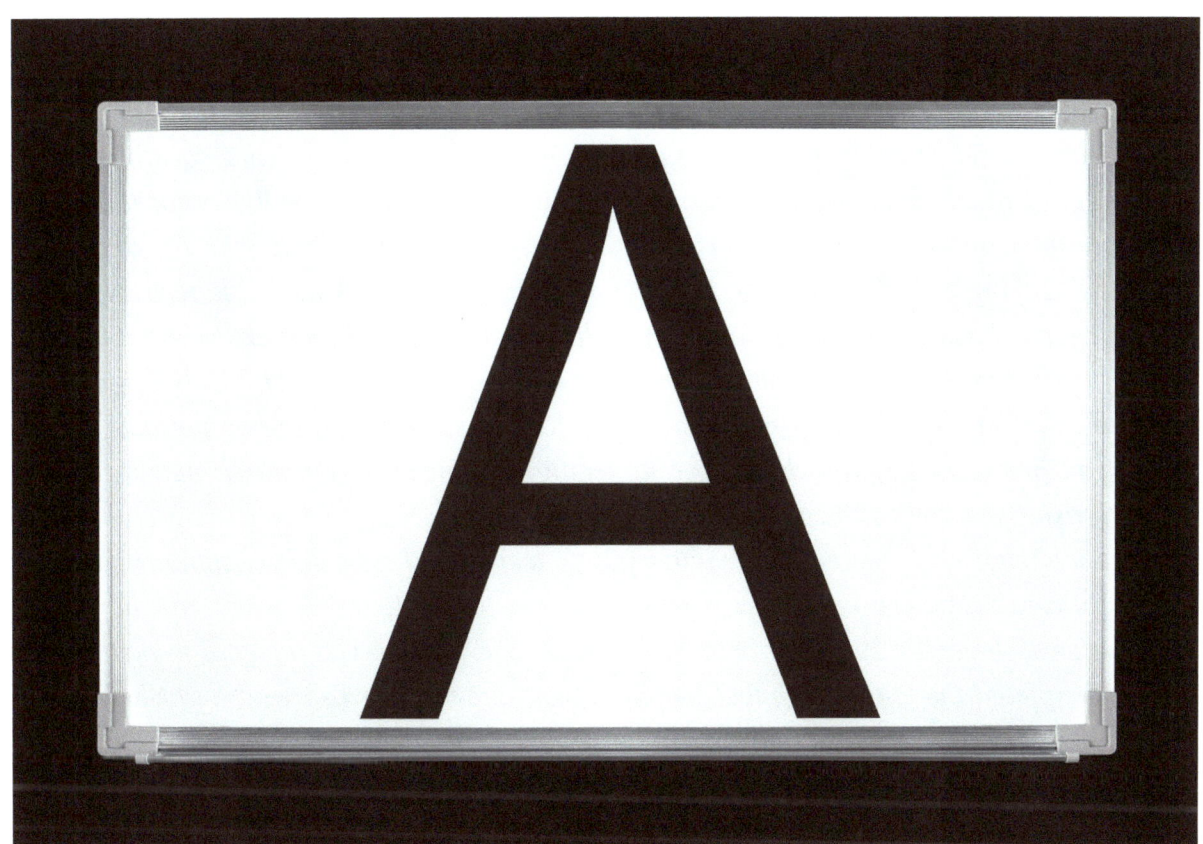

Close your eyes tight, and Imagine an Erasable Whiteboard right in front of you within arm's reach. Continue to see it in your mind's eye. And if you cannot see it, imagine that you do.

Now notice, at the bottom of the Whiteboard, there is a rail, and on the rail is an eraser and a Black colored erasable marker. In the center of the Whiteboard there is a large Letter A drawn with the marker. The A almost touches the frame at all three points or ends of the A. What I would like you to do is to imagine yourself erasing the letter A but before you do, I want to make sure that you don't touch the frame while erasing the letter A So, what I would like you to do is to first, make a small break at each end of the A where it touches the frame. When you are done,

*.....you'll notice that the A is separated from the frame so that you can erase the letter A without touching the frame in any way......Now visualize that you are looking at yourself from behind watching yourself picking up the eraser and erasing the letter A. Do it now, and do it carefully (pause)Very good. Now Watching yourself,... start with the letter A again, (the letters can be capitalized or lower case) and make the letter A on the-Whiteboard like the A was drawn, almost touching the frame. Now, erase just the points where the letter A almost touches the frame then, completely Erase the letter A. Continue with the letter **B, in the same manner,** making the letter **B** and carefully erasing the almost touching points and then completely erasing the letter **B.** do not touch the frame in any way while making or erasing the letters. Now...Continue with the alphabet, You'll be hearing me, But **Your job** is to very carefully keep making the letters and erasing the letters Through to Z continuing on with the letter **C** and then erase the letter **C** ...**Each** time you make a letter, and each time you erase a letter, you will go deeper and deeper into a narrowing of your consciousness,concentrating on nothing but the letter you are working with, hearing and seeing nothing else. Continue making a letter and erasing a letter you begin to relax more and more so very relaxed--Just continue to make each letter and then erase the letter going deeper and even deeper into relaxation-so very relaxed very very relaxed-and when you get to the letter Z, when you have made and erased the entire alphabet, you will raise your right hand as a signal to me that you have completed the entire alphabet but when you attempt to raise your right hand, it **will** feel very very heavy,almost like I am holding your arm down, it is Soooooooo heavy but TRY to raise it again just a slight movement will be enough...................OK relax..*

Now, the weight is gone and you can raise your arm effortlessly as if it is floating...

Your client can now listen and receive helpful and beneficial suggestions.

Suggestions

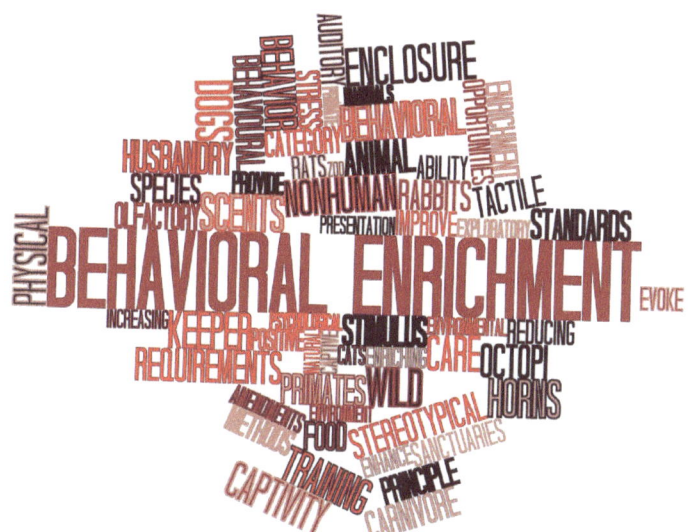

Seriate; A more accurately descriptive, up to date term for Post Hypnotic would be
<u>SERIATE SUGGESTIONS</u>

The value and objective of Hypnosis is that **a suggestion given in Hypnosis** *will be carried out later, in a conscious state and by constant repetition (conditioning), become a permanent response or behavior*

Positive Suggestion Management

The Most effective Hypnotic suggestions are "replacements" the basis of Hypnosis. Is suggestion. The Hypnotist should not simply tell a client who is afraid of flying, "You are no longer afraid of flying." Instead, the Hypnotist should suggest that the patient imagine how wonderful it feels to be riding in an airplane, and how much safer it is than traveling in a in a car. To a patient about to undergo a painful procedure the Hypnotist does not say, "This won't hurt a bit." Instead, the Hypnotist should suggest that the patient experience the pain as a feeling of warmth or pressure.

Because therapists do not know which ideas will be best received by any patient, they utilize an assortment of suggestions and metaphors. A person afraid of public speaking might be told, for example, to focus on before getting up to speak that the audience is a group of close personal friends or that they are all convinced that he is the most respected expert in the subject matter he is presenting....

Criteria: For Effective Hypnosis suggestions

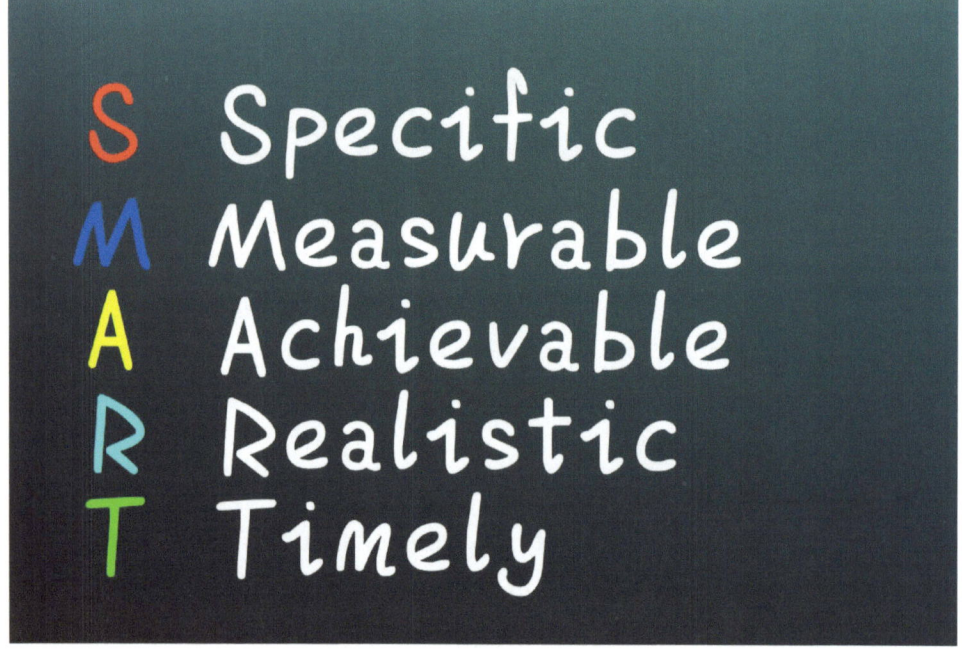

Positive concepts
Simple, short sentences
Believable
Measurable.....

Deepening Suggestions

A Hypnotic suggestion is a suggestion given in Hypnosis that will be acted on when not in Hypnosis.

Tell each subject,

(especially in the first session), *"The next time you go into Hypnosis, you will go into Hypnosis much more readily, and also much, much, deeper"!*

Subliminal Deepening The use Computer generated subliminal audio deepening suggestions during the deepening phase of Induction is a very powerful modern deepening technique.

Feedback

Create imaginary scenes for the subjects involving all the senses. Such as a canoe ride in a shallow lake with their arm dragging in the cold water. Create a scenario. Hear the birds in the trees. Smell the roses. Feel the warmth of the sun, feel the cool breezes, etc. After the session, question the subject as to which senses were most involved. Then in the next sessions, use those senses for deepening Hypnosis

Repeated Audio Visual Subliminal Inductions
(This may not be legal in some jurisdictions, Check your local laws.)

Immediate additional inductions within the same session will result in deepening past stage 3

During a single session; Hypnotize, give suggestions, have the subject open their eyes in Hypnosis for subliminal Video impressions and then close their eyes again and repeat the audio suggestions.

Counting Backwards *"As I count backwards from 50 to 1, you will go deeper, 50.....deeper and deeper, 49..... all the way down deep.......etc."* This is a very simple method and effective.

If You must leave the room with the subject in Hypnosis, Tell the subject that you are going to leave the room for a minute and instruct them to: *"Count mentally from 100 - 1, and as you do, you will go deeper and deeper into Hypnosis".*

Seriate (*After Hypnosis*) and *in Session responses* to suggestions

<u>*Hypnotically induced reactions are the essence of the art and a very serious responsibility assumed by the Hypnotist-Practitioner*</u>

A number is suggested to be forgotten in Hypnosis,
It will, but this effect will fade rapidly Post Hypnosis

A conscious response
Such as one triggered by **a signal** induced during the Hypnotic session such as by a doctor or practitioner touching a subject's shoulder and telling the subject that they will then close their eyes and relax.

Analgesia can be induced At level 4,
In a dental procedure, where Hypnotic, analgesia is induced in the subjects jaw and the subject is told that they will remain in this condition until The dentist taps on their jaw twice. A tooth could be extracted painlessly.

RE:De Pascalis, V.; Magurano, M.R.; Bellusci, A. (1999). "Pain perception, event-related potentials and skin conductance responses to painful"stimuli in high, mid, and low hypnotizable subjects: Effects of differential pain reduction strategies"

This effect will gradually wear off...**Analgesia may not be legal in some states Check <u>your local laws.</u>**

SCRIPTS:

Progressive Relaxation

Is primarily employed as a versatile master induction procedure.

Generic **INDUCTION**

to Level 3, using personalized Progressive Relaxation

Copyright 09/01/20010 revised 01/13/2013 By H.L.Silvia,M Ch Ph.D Palm Beach Hypnosis Institute

Subliminals should be added separately

001A....*Client's Name............,* You are About to Participate in a relaxing refreshing and very beneficial experience

001B-- *Now.,* keeping your head level Look straight ahead , ….OK,…now… moving only your eyes look up, as high as you can and pick out a spot to focus on…….Keep looking up …hold that spot as I talk to you….keep looking up…as I count to 10 … 1-2 etc., it is difficult to keep looking up but concentrate on that spot………Your eyelids are becoming very tired and heavy but keep looking up…. holding that spot…..it is very difficult keep your eyes up …......................Now slowly…..Close your eyes and relax

001c

…. In a moment I will ask you to Take 6 Very Deep and Rapid inhaling and exhaling, Cleansing Breaths, OK first, inhale deeply and fully as possible and then…… Exhale Forcefully and completely. do this 5 mort times---- , 3, 4, 5, 6, Now Relax….

You are now breathing deeply and comfortably, a feeling of total relaxation is spreading Throughout… your body…….. And as we continue to talk…..You will make small automatic unconscious adjustments to suit your comfort

Zzz

001d

.…We will…Now concentrate on relaxing your whole body one part at a time You will begin to relax to allow yourself to enter and experience that comfortable, peaceful state of mind that you feel just before you go to sleep. Where WE can access and influence your subconscious memory…..

002A *Relaxation*

Now ……… RE….L…AX ALL those muscle groups around your face…………. This is just a start, ….notice how your whole face feels as if it is softening…..

ttttttttttttttttttttttttttttttttttttttttttttttttttttttttttttttttttttttttttt

…RELAX your scalp……..Notice how this is RE….LAX ING your forehead..and this feeling is flowing down to your eyebrows.……..and now…..Your eyelids…..Now this sensation is spreading to your cheeks….it is Releasing the tension around your nose and your mouth….. Your lips feel Soft and they are starting to RELAX……

ttttttttt, Your Jaw is now loose and relaxed …..along with all those muscle groups of your face….. just RE…..LAX..ing…..

You are ……….Just…….. letting go now………ttttttttttttttttttttttttttttttttttttttttzzzzzzzzzzzzz

……..You can feel the front part of your neck Relaxing…., let your head drop loosely forward, this will relax the back part of your neck…. now just roll your head lightly, side to side, …...releasing any tension ….

Feel your shoulders just starting to RELAX….Make a light shrug, which will let go any tension that may be in your shoulder area……

tttttttttttttttttttttttttttttttttttttttttttttttttttttttttttttttttttttttttttttttt
ttttttttttttttttttttttttttttttttttttttttttt

…IT feels so good to just RE…L..AX..

……. Your upper arms are relaxing……..This soft warm feeling is flowing down from your shoulder area and around your elbows through to your forearms……….It is Relaxing your wrists……. and now…….. your hands….. …….even your fingers are now completely relaxed...

ttttttttttttttttttttttttttttttttttttttttttttttttttttttttttttttttttttttttttttttt

77

Your arms feel very heavy….but relaxed…..A Comforting, Warm, Moist, Heavy towel has been laid on each of them…………, …….Notice how much deeper and regular your breathing has become………………You are Feeling the comfortable soothing natural relaxed rhythm of your breathing……… …. When you exhale, You Allow all your chest muscles to RELAX completely……..allll…….. the way down, relaxing your stomach muscles……………Now, There is a soft warm relaxed feeling in your stomach area…….zzzzzzzzzzzzzzzz…..It feels so good to just RE…L.AX……. zzzzzzzz Allow your back muscles to RE..L…AX…….those large muscle groups in the upper part of your back…….Now allow that warm smooth feeling to flow down your spine and into your lower back…..just…….. Re…..lax……

…. This wonderful flow of relaxation is flowing around Your hips ….. down around and through to your thighs….It is RE..LAXing your thighs…..and flowing smoothly around your knees……… to your legs, …. Re…lax..ing your calves….and your ankles…….RE…LAX.ing your feet………. even your TOES are now completely Re…laxed………….. Now…………. just allow yourself to enjoy and bask in this warm safe soothing state as you begin to go into a very deep and Comfortable state…………….feeling so goooood……. and completely

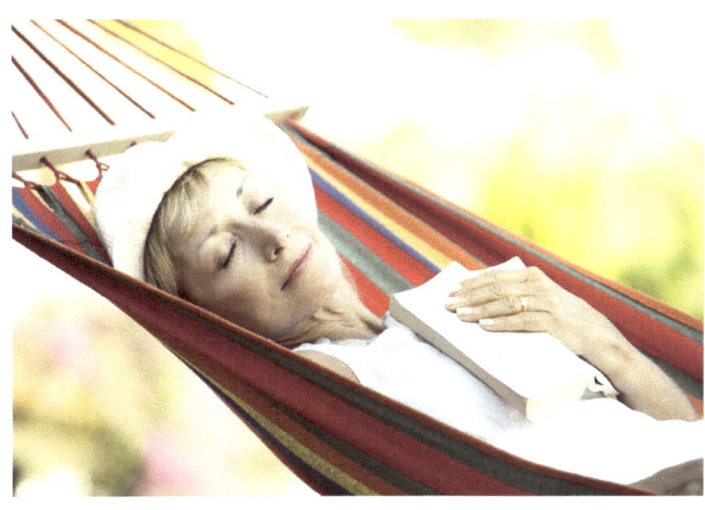

Relaxed. …..PAUSE ………………………………………

002b ....You will experience some sort of feelings as you go into this deep relaxed *state*. Possibly a slight numbness …… usually in your arms …….

(Not at stage 2 yet)

You may experience a comfortable floating sensation or a lightness in Your Body…..........enjoy it

ttttttttttttttttttttttttttttttttttttttttttttttttttttttttttttttttttttttttttttttttt

…………………..You may also notice that when you just let go and totally relax You may need to swallow…….go ahead, that's normal, your saliva glands have a tendency to relax while in this state……

When You just start to let go and totally relax, ….Your eyes relax and you will see tiny very light pinpoints of light…..its a comfortable feeling….like laying in a quiet peaceful summer meadow at night and watching the stars……

ttttttttttttttttttttttttttttttttttttttttttttttttttttttttttttttttttttttttttttttttt

……ALL these things are positive, beneficial benefits of your just letting go and relaxing……..The important thing is that these sensations represent and indicate your *WILLINGNESS, and your READINESS*…. to ALLOW yourself to go into *Hypnosis*……….Going into Hypnosis is soothing and gradual, experience.

003A *Into Hypnosis*

††

Now Just imagine you are resting on a summer night in that quiet peaceful meadow on a very comfortable soft cloud like cushion that is shaped to fit your body and..........

that...Time and distance have no meaning…….. You are able to ride on that cloud safely, smoothly and quietly to…….Your Place That special place in your life,…. a place where you were Very content , calm, SAFE and serene..........

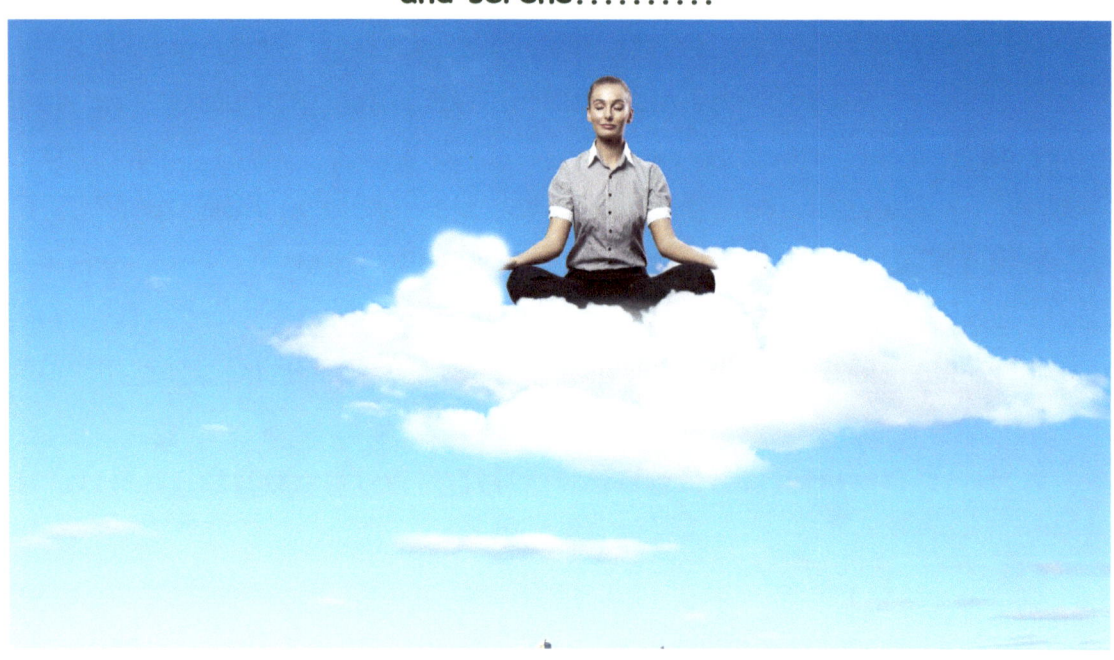

……….Allow your cloud to take you there, Now…... .
Going softly,…………………….. You are there...content, safe, and relaxed.
Stay and savor that place ……..
(***30 sec. pause)
T††
††††††††††††††††††††††††††††††

003b…………..Now Comfortably.. but… Deeply inhale,..1 2 3 4…….. and……
Exhale 1-2-3.4……. comfortably,….

☨☨☨
☨☨☨☨☨☨☨☨☨☨☨☨☨☨☨☨☨☨☨☨

As I begin to count again-You will go deeper and deeper into Hypnosis… and on each count, you will ALLOW yourself to drift further into Hypnosis. Any outside noise or sounds will reinforce the strength of the count guiding you into an increasingly comfortable state of Deep Hypnosis.

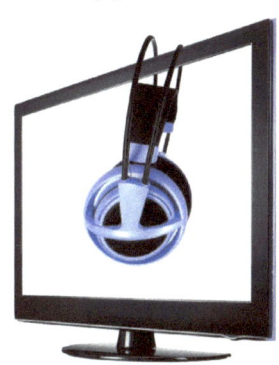

1…….DEEEPER and DEEPER……..now…..2, ALLLL…..the way down…..DEEPER…..3…..4…..tired and drowsy…..5…..6…..just letting go…..Now….7….8…..DEEPER………..AND………..DEEPER…..9…..You are relaxed and letting go…..10…..11…..12….. ????? ALLLL the way down………..DEEPER…..and…..DEEPER…..19..AND 20…..DEEPER Into A beautifully quiet, serene, Meditative State …..Awareness of your inner self ……….003c…<u>Add Subliminal Visual reinforcement here</u>

Now, you are in a deep state of Hypnosis, slowly open your eyes and let yourself focus on nothing but the beautiful calming interesting image directly in front of you.

Relax and allow the beneficial suggestions and Ideas to come gently to you. They will stay with your subconscious and enhance your well being long after this session is over (1 min +++visual and audio Subliminals) .Now Slowly close your eyes.

004A Convincer-Reinforcement

Your arms are very heavy,…. Remember those heavy warm soothing towels softly laid on them……..Your arms are so heavy that it is very difficult to move or lift them ………accept this soothing feeling …just for now…….

Zzzzzzzzzzzzzzzzzzzzzzzzzzzzzzzzzzzzzzzzzzzzzzz

005A-6A:::(Foundation for and Suggestions)

Your mind is now RELAXED and open to receive More *HELPFUL* and BENEFICIAL COMMANDS that I am about to give you.

005b VISUALIZE YOURSELF relaxing on your cloud like Chair, ("Your Place"), looking down at your body which is reclining about 6 feet away where you started this experience,

Notice that You can feel comfortably, totally detached,

But now you realize the actual You,…..(Your Mind)

is separate…. ……………...and in command of your body.

006….Basic Suggestions:::

006b PBHI Basic Suggestion 001…………………..You are now aware of your powerful ability to relax and enter this state of detachment… Your real inner self

You are completely comfortable and in control….without any discomfort or distracting sensations sounds or thoughts… Now,…………… You are in control

006c PBHI Suggestion 002…..…….. Remember After you Leave this session ….You can return to your Special Private Place by Taking A *very* deep breath, Clenching your downward facing right fist, then as you exhale, turn your hand upward while opening your hand and saying to yourself…… "MY PLACE."

006d PBHI Suggestion 003…. Every time you access and enter…<u>Your</u> Special Private place and look with comfortable detachment at your body… you will find that,… At will,…. You can (with practice) in this state, control any sensations and functions you formerly thought were automatic…. …. You are in control… You can Recall useful wonderful memories, beneficial thoughts and actions stored in your subconscious ……..You will realize that this is a perfect state of meditation…..

OR…….. Custom, Client's COMMANDS HERE:

:

Then:
007 Exit Awakening / Exit Script:

..........In a moment I am going to count from one to five and on the count of five and you will open your eyes feeling wonderful in every way.

1....Coming out of Hypnosis, You are feeling wonderful.. in every way.....

2...You are continuing to emerge now from Hypnosis....... feeling wonderful in every way........... and it will be much easier for you to go back into Hypnosis the next time.....

3.You.........remember the helpful and beneficial suggestions...

4.You are..........Starting to come back now...and ....

5 ...." You are ……. OUT OF HYPNOSIS NOW, YOUR EYES ARE WIDE OPEN, YOU ARE FEELING WONDERFULLY REFRESHED AND ALERT...

After awakening, the subject will still be receptive to suggestions and instructions such as:

...Wasn't that wonderful??? Don't you feel so much better now?

Every time you go into Hypnosis it becomes Easier and more effective.

If your your Pulse and blood Pressure were to be taken now both would be significantly lower and closer to your ideal state

You can Go to your place as often as you want, but the best times are

1. Before you get out of bed in the morning
2. After Lunch
3. In bed in the evening, just before sleep…… BUT!

DO NOT DRIVE OR OPERATE MACHINERY FOR AT LEAST 15 MINUTES

Copyright 09/01/20010 revised 01/13/2013 By H.L.Silvia,MCH PhD Palm Beach Hypnosis Institute
Copyright is granted solely to Certified student graduates of courses offered by the Palm Beach Hypnosis Institute llc

Understanding The Freedom from Nicotine addiction series

Stop Smoking Commands .©2008 Palm Beach Hypnosis Institute

The human mind and body can be superficially described as a magnificently efficient, automatically operating chemical and electrical system... Which You have the *option to control*

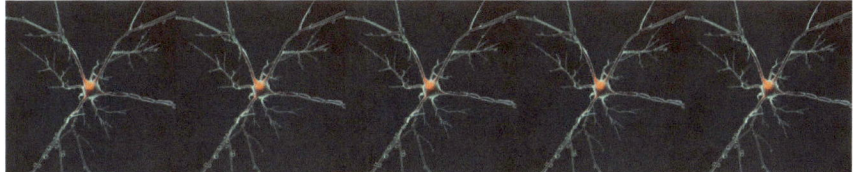

Visualize these 5 nerve endings and their receptors in your brain.

These are the connections to your body's wonderful, complete, ever adapting and growing automatic operating system.(The Autonomous Nervous System). Each connection has a receptor and sensor specifically shaped like a keyhole and key to receive or send a special chemical molecule which can be a stimulus or signal necessary to operate your body... signaling a need or a signal for instance, to increase or decrease your heartbeat....or Blood pressure...

When we ingest substitute chemicals that stimulate these connections, sooner or later, the connections alter to accept only those substitutes, the brain connections no longer demand our body to manufacture of its own natural product......

Smoking, or any use of Nicotine, is an example....It is an imperfect substitute for our natural, automatically occurring chemical substances.

You will feel Your Heart rate increase, notice Your blood pressure going up. Your arteries will constrict making the heart work harder. After smoking for enough time to condition and alter those vital operating connections in the brain with imperfect substitutes,

The effect of introducing artificial operating chemicals decreases the production of your natural substances.

We will, in your deeply relaxed Hypnotic state, *Gradually* block the artificially created nicotine receptors, Your system will *Gradually* create and supply its own natural Endomorphins and supplements.

Imagine yourself at age 10, free of all the unnecessary ingested mood, mind, and body altering chemicals which later impeded or sidetracked your full potential for growth and enjoyment...That state is still attainable....

A fresh start.

In the course of 5 sessions, approximately 1 hour each, We will use the Hypnotic state

to directly address and direct your Body's Subconscious Autonomic system to

accept beneficial commands and modifications. Then, we will give you the simple

equipment and instructions for continually reinforcing your freedom from nicotine.

Guaranteed for life, You may return for the complete treatment regime anytime after 30 days from your last appointment...©2008 Palm Beach Hypnosis Institute

The palm beach Hypnosis Institute grants the copyright and use of this session to Certified Students of its Training courses

STOP SMOKING COMMANDS-SESSION ONE ©
©2008 Palm Beach Hypnosis Institute

You are completely and Totally relaxed and ready to receive exact beneficial commands which you will use to replace your desire for nicotine with a warm comfortable, relaxed, feeling anytime you wish.

The conscious desire for nicotine is simply a response to a chemical demand signal, which you can erase and then direct your natural internal system to operate in a very desirable and beneficial way.

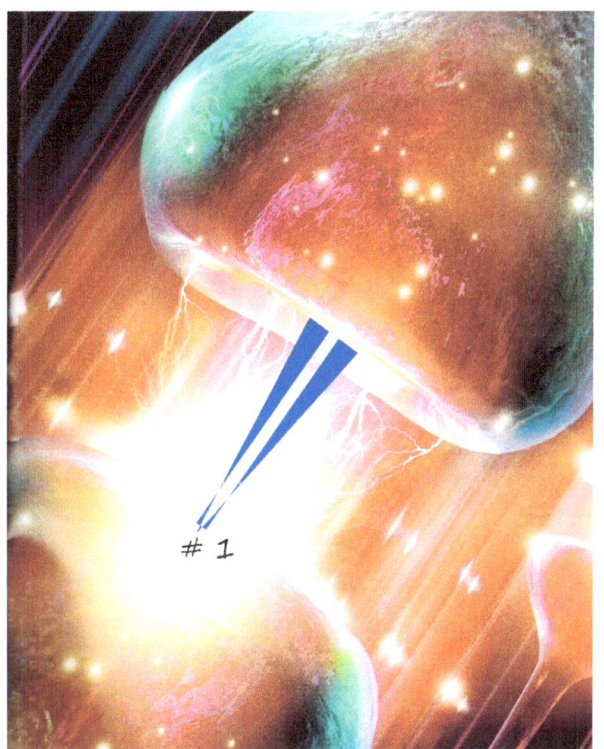

Visualize With your mind's eye the internal, front section of your brain containing the Five, microscopic, nerve junctions, that have been artificially shaped by Nicotine to accept the Nicotine molecules. Mentally Create an intense cold blue microscopic beam and direct it to the first receptor, naming it ..(#1).... now erase the tiny nicotine molecule shaped indentations in that receptor with the beam, leaving it smooth and empty ..

Now, let your natural system re-create a Warm Golden, Natural Relaxing endorphin...Guide it into the empty #1 receptor.

This has reduced your conscious desire for nicotine by One Fifth......Enough, along with a strong conscious effort, to reduce your nicotine demand for 24hours...You **will** notice, After fully awakening from this Hypnosis session, and upon Your first attempt to count from one to ten, You will have a very strong desire to use the

LATIN word OCHO for the ENGLISH number EIGHT

....and You also will find that your blood pressure and heart rate have decreased significantly

Smoking exit (After each session's commands)
You have been given EXACT BENEFICIAL commands...
In a moment I am going to count from one to five and on the count of five you will open your eyes feeling wonderful in every way..........
ONE...You are Coming out of Hypnosis, and you feel wonderful in every way... Your unconscious desire for nicotine has been reduced by one fifth,(20%)
TWO.......You are Continuing to emerge from Hypnosis, feeling wonderful in every way. It will be much easier and you will be more eager to go into Hypnosis the next time.....
THREE........Remember those Helpful, EXACT and BENEFICIAL suggestions......You are Starting to come back now...........and........
Notice the intentionally absent # 4 ???
FIVE ...YOU are out of Hypnosis now, Your eyes are wide open, You are feeling refreshed and
ALERT!

STOP SMOKING COMMANDS-SESSION TWO ©
©2008 Palm Beach Hypnosis Institute

You are completely and Totally relaxed and ready to receive exact beneficial commands which you will use to achieve your desired objectives...

The conscious desire to smoke is simply a response to a chemical demand signal for Nicotine, which you have already, Partially erased to let your natural internal system operate in its most beneficial way......

With your mind's eye, Again, Visualize the internal front section of your brain containing the remaining FOUR, microscopic, nerve junctions, artificially shaped to accept the Nicotine Molecules---

Mentally Create an intense cold blue microscopic dot and direct it to the SECOND receptor,(#2) and watch the tiny indentations representing the nicotine molecule smooth out leaving an empty receptor

Now, allow your natural system create a Warm Golden, Soothing, Natural endorphin molecule. Guide it into the empty #2 receptor.

This has reduced your conscious desire for Nicotine by TWO FIFTHS .... Enough, along with a mild Conscious effort, to function comfortably without nicotine for another 24 hours............or longer

After fully awakening from this Hypnosis session, Upon Your FIRST attempt to count from one to ten,...................
You will have an impulse use the LATIN word DOS for the ENGLISH number TWO

Later, after you return to a fully awakened state, you will find that your blood pressure and heart rate have again, decreased significantly.

The palm beach Hypnosis Institute grants the copyright and use of this session to Certified Students of its Training courses

STOP SMOKING COMMANDS-SESSION THREE ©

©2008 Palm Beach Hypnosis Institute

You are completely and Totally relaxed and ready to receive exact beneficial commands which you will use to achieve your desired objectives...

The conscious desire to smoke is simply a response to a chemical demand signal for Nicotine, which you are gradually erasing to let your natural internal system operate in its most beneficial way......

With your mind's eye, Again, Visualize the internal front section of your brain containing the remaining THREE, microscopic, artificially shaped keyhole-like receptors for Nicotine.

Mentally Re-Create That intense cold blue microscopic dot and direct it to the THIRD receptor,(#3) and watch the tiny indentations representing the nicotine molecule smooth out leaving an empty receptor

Now, allow your natural system create a Warm Relaxing Golden, flow of Natural Endorphins................Guide it all into the empty #3 receptor.

This has replaced your system's requirement for Nicotine by THREE FIFTHS ... Enough, to be <u>almost</u> completely free of any chemical signal for Nicotine....

After fully awakening from this Hypnosis session, and Upon Your FIRST attempt to count from one to ten, You will want to and will probably use the Latin word ....TRES for the ENGLISH number THREE

Later, after you return to a fully awakened state, you will find that your blood pressure and heart rate have again decreased significantly and you will feel unusually relaxed and comfortable..You have been given some very EXACT BENEFICIAL commands.

In a moment I am going to count from one to five and on the count of five you will open your eyes, feeling wonderful and relaxed in every way..........etc

STOP SMOKING COMMANDS-SESSION FOUR©
©2008 Palm Beach Hypnosis Institute

You are completely and Totally relaxed and ready to receive exact beneficial commands which you will use to achieve your desired objectives...

The conscious desire to smoke is simply a response to a chemical demand signal for Nicotine, which you have been erasing to let your natural internal system operate in its most beneficial way......

You Now can effortlessly Visualize the internal front section of your brain containing your remaining TWO, Microscopic, nerve junctions, artificially shaped to accept the Nicotine Molecules---

Create that intense cold blue microscopic dot and direct it to the FOURTH receptor,(#4) and erase the tiny indentations shaped to accept the nicotine molecules.

Now, allow your natural system summon a Warm Relaxing Golden, flow of Natural Endorphins and Guide it all into the empty #3 receptor.

This has replaced your conscious and unconscious requirement for Nicotine by FOUR FIFTHS .... and created a sensation of mild euphoria Smoking no longer is necessary ....

After fully awakening from this Hypnosis session, Upon Your FIRST attempt to count from one to ten, You will want to use the LATIN word QUATRO for the ENGLISH number FOUR......it is OK to resist that impulse.

Later, after you return to a fully awakened state, you will want to tell others about this wonderful and serene state that you can invoke any time you wish.

The palm beach Hypnosis Institute grants the copyright and use of this session to Certified Students of its Training courses

STOP SMOKING COMMANDS-SESSION (Final) FIVE
©2008 Palm Beach Hypnosis Institute

You are completely and Totally relaxed and ready to receive the FINAL exact beneficial commands which you will use to achieve your COMPLETE freedom from your former artificially induced desire for Nicotine

You now have experienced and understand that under Hypnosis, you can direct your Mind-Body Control system to replace the chemical demand signal for Nicotine With natural internally created soothing, Endomorphins………
TODAY IS SPECIAL…...Mark the Date on your calendar…

FINALLY……While Visualizing the internal front section of your brain containing the LAST, microscopic, nerve junction that is still artificially shaped to accept the Nicotine Molecules, #5………………………..

Mentally Re-Energize Your intense cold blue microscopic Beam and direct it to the LAST receptor(#5)… and watch the tiny indentations representing the nicotine molecule smooth out, leaving an empty receptor.

Again, allow your natural system create a Warm Golden, Natural Relaxing flow of Natural Endomorphins ……………Guide into that empty, Last, (#5) receptor ' You are now experiencing a feeling of well being and relief… a naturally induced state of mild euphoria

You have REMOVED the Artificially induced apparent desire for Nicotine and Replaced it with a set of receptors that can accept Soothing Natural Endorphins which you can now summon at will to produce a feeling of relaxation and Well being……..

From this moment on, anytime you wish to create that flow of beneficial relaxing refreshing Endomorphins, all you have to do is take 5 deep, comfortable, slow breaths, while repeating mentally, "GOLDEN" with each exhaling breath and enjoy that feeling of refreshing relaxation that this command will create.

Upon fully awakening from this Hypnosis session, and Upon Your FIRST attempt to count from one to ten, You will instead of the number THREE you may exclaim, if you wish…… "FREE AT LAST"

You have developed a new and powerful skill
Share this accomplishment with special people,
Let the OTHERS wonder.

After you return to a fully awakened state, your blood pressure and heart rate
WILL BE MORE ACCEPTABLE THAN THEY HAVE BEEN FOR YEARS ………
and your ability to take a deep refreshing breath without hesitation has returned.

You have been given and executed EXACT BENEFICIAL commands.

In a moment I am going to count from one to five and on the count of five you will open your eyes feeling a new freedom and wonderful in every way……….

ONE………….You are Coming out of Hypnosis, feeling a new freedom and feeling more
wonderful in every way

TWO…….continuing to emerge now from Hypnosis feeling a new freedom and wonderful in every way.

THREE…….. It is now very easy to go into self Hypnosis to reinforce this new freedom All you have to do is take 5 deep, comfortable, slow breaths, while repeating mentally, **"Golden"** with each exhaling breath and enjoy that feeling of refreshing relaxation That this command will create. It has been intensely re-enforced subliminally into your unconscious

FOUR Starting to come back now………..and……..

FIVE ……Out of Hypnosis now, your eyes are wide open and you are feeling refreshed and alert
Take a slow comfortable deep breath, Exhale slowly.

"Golden" has been intensely reinforced subliminally into your unconscious.

Nicotine-end of series commentary:

This session has been strengthened with intense subliminal, (below your threshold of conscious perception), suggestions, statements, commands and other proprietaries.

When *experienced during* the day it will result in a highly relaxed state of mind and body.

Do not, absolutely, do not attempt to drive or operate any machinery for at least 15 minutes after each session...

Success with This 5 day series is dependent upon your commitment to play the reinforcement session each day before leaving bed in the morning, again immediately after your mid-day meal, immediately after dinner and lastly in bed before you go to sleep...

Usually after the 3rd day you may go to a state of full somnambulistic Hypnosis during the evening session. That is normal. You will either wake up at the end or simply drift into an noticeably comfortable full night's sleep.......

Repetition is essential...

For Three weeks listen to and participate in the reinforcement audio three times each day.

First-in the morning in bed

Second-after your mid day meal

Third-in bed, for a wonderful night's rest

At this point instruct the client in the Palm Beach Hypnosis Institutes's Proprietary reinforcement modality.

No longer a Smoker,
Daily Reinforcement session ©

©2008 Palm Beach Hypnosis Institute

Record this session and give it to the client with the instruction to play back at least three times each day for 30 days

You are completely and Totally relaxed and ready to create strong beneficial natural soothing Endomorphins which you will use regularly to maintain your COMPLETE freedom from your former artificially induced desire for Nicotine. You now have experienced and understand that under Hypnosis, you can direct your Mind-Body Control system to again Create internally, natural soothing, Endomorphins……and experience a feeling of well being and relief……

YOU have Totally restored those artificially altered receptors to a natural state and

REMOVED the Artificially induced apparent desire for Nicotine and Replaced it with a set of receptors that can accept Soothing Natural Endorphins which you can summon at will to produce a feeling of relaxation and Well being……..From this moment on, To summon those beneficial relaxing refreshing Endorphins at will, All you have to do is take 5 rapid deep, breaths, while repeating mentally, "Golden" with each exhaling breath to enjoy that feeling of refreshing relaxation That this command will give you. It has been intensely reinforced subliminally into your unconscious. You have developed a new and powerful skill

Share this accomplishment with special people,

and let the rest wonder.

Printed reinforcement instructions for the client.

This session has been strongly reinforced by intense subliminal, (below your threshold of conscious Perception), statements, suggestions and commands. and other proprietaries. When *experienced during* the day it will result in a highly relaxed state of mind and body.

Do not, absolutely, do not attempt to drive or operate any machinery for at least 15 minutes after each session...

Success with This 5 day series is dependent upon your commitment to play the reinforcement session before leaving bed in the morning, again immediately after your mid-day meal, immediately after dinner and optionaly, in bed before you go to sleep...

Usually after the 3rd in clinic day you may go to a state of full somnambulistic Hypnosis during the evening session. That is normal. You will either wake up at the end or simply drift into an noticeably comfortable full night's sleep......

Repetition is essential...

Awakening

When awakening, the following language should be used in the first session "......In a moment, I'm going to count from one to five, and on the count of five you will open your eyes feeling wonderful in every way. *1*...coming out of Hypnosis, feeling wonderful in every way.....*2*...You are continuing to emerge now from Hypnosis, You are feeling wonderful in every way. It will be that much easier for you to go back into Hypnosis the next time......*3*.....remember the helpful and beneficial suggestions....*4* You are starting to come back now.....and

5....,You are ....OUT of Hypnosis now, Your eyes are wide open, and you are feeling wonderfully refreshed and relaxed!"

Always make notes of sensations and impressions to customize subsequent sessions.

Ask your client to describe with as much detail as they can, what they experienced, and record their impressions and sensations regarding Time distortion, numbness, tingling, heaviness, etc. The sensations can be exploited in the next session to trigger Hypnosis.

Reinforcement of the Hypnotic experience

Once your client has experienced their first Hypnosis session, regardless of the depth level you have induced, the client's response to suggestions and experiences in subsequent sessions will be intensified.

To Deepen or continue to intensify the effectiveness within each session you may employ:

Pyramiding By bringing the subject out of Hypnosis and immediately repeating the induction 2 or more times.

Convincers During the session, demonstrate to the subject sensations of heat and cold that they are experiencing, or the cataleptic inability to raise an arm even simple catalepsy, such as rotating one hand so that the palm is facing up. These experiences will deepen the trance and the receptiveness of your subject.

Daily Self Reinforcement

A Recording of the session or a custom, specifically created, computer enhanced, *Reinforcement* file for the client to apply on a daily basis will create a more cost effective and more convenient experience for the client.

Research and Modern Technology Has provided us with variety of very effective psychoactive audio and Subliminal image equipment and software with which can induce specific moods and emotions with the selection of specific volume, frequency, tones, colors and images.

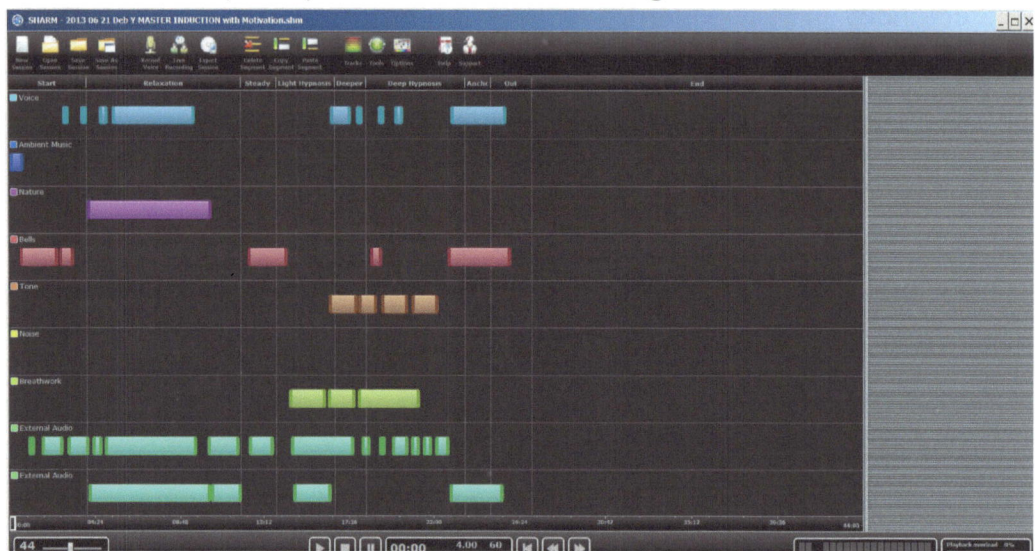

Here, at the Florida Holistics Institute we offer the _graduates of this course_ Additional short Sessions in applied computer software and equipment used effectively at The Palm Beach Hypnosis Institute. SharmScreen1.jpg

CHAPTER FOUR
SELF Hypnosis

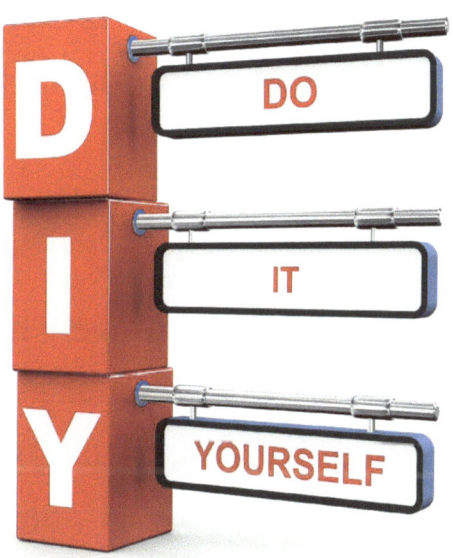

A 3 Step Method

Step 1..... Pre-sleep

Starting tonight; just before you are ready to fall asleep, say to yourself
10 times:

> *"Every day in every way, I am becoming better and better "*.

Do not allow yourself to fall asleep and lose count. Every time you say this suggestion hold each finger of your right hand with your left hand, Then

1. change over and hold each finger of your right hand until you've completed the suggestion 10 times. This will be your first real experience in effectively programming yourself through suggestion. It is necessary to accomplish this exercise *every* night without falling asleep until you have completed the 10 repetitions, establishing a habit pattern of effectively programming yourself with positive, useful suggestions before going to sleep. Soon, you will realize that the suggestion is very positively influencing your daily life and attitude.

Step 2

Induction

Continue with step 1, the before-sleep technique......for 1 week.

   Now, twice each day, in the morning and in the evening you will Hypnotize yourself and stay in Hypnosis for 2-3 minutes, and then take yourself out:

Sit or recline in a comfortable chair.

While focusing your attention effortlessly on a spot opposite you just a little above eye level,

take *three* slow deep breaths and as you inhale your *third* breath, hold it for *three* full seconds. then........close your eyes, exhale, relax and allow yourself to go into a deep sound Hypnotic rest.

You will remain in Hypnosis for approximately two to three minutes by slowly counting backwards from 100 to one, picturing each number in your favorite color on a Large, up close, TV screen as you count. To awaken, just count forward one, two, and three, and open your eyes, You will feel Refreshed and alert.

Do this twice a day for 7 days after which time you will be ready for the third and final step of self-Hypnosis.

Step 3

The Programmed Suggestion

This third step in self Hypnosis is to be started one week after you complete the exercises for step 2. ..... **Now discontinue 2.**

For step 3, Using a business card, which you can easily carry with you at all times. Write the suggestion you've prepared for yourself which meets the criteria of being positive, simple and believable as well as measurable.

Always state your suggestion in the present tense.

You may use your Smart-phone, record this suggestion three times and save it.

Now you may relax and choose a spot opposite you, slightly above eye level. Hold the card in front of the spot and read the suggestion to yourself 3 times **or** plug in your ear-buds, close your eyes and listen to your recording and allow yourself to imagine accomplishing what is stated. UNLEASH your imagination!!

You've and written your suggestion on a card, recorded it and chosen your spot, read or played the suggestion to yourself three times. Now, take your first deep breath. Exhale. Take your second deep breath. Exhale. Now, take your third deep breath and hold it, close your eyes and count backward from three to one. Exhale and go deep into Hypnosis. At this point, instead of counting backward from 100 to 1, allow the suggestion to repeat over and over in your subconscious mind.

Let your subconscious mind see you carrying out your suggestion.

You'll find that at times the words start to break up and become fragmented. That's perfectly alright. The important words or phrases will come through to you.

In approximately two to three minutes you'll have a feeling that it's time to stop and come out. At this point, just count forward, one....two....three and open your eyes. You will feel refreshed, alert, and ready to go.

Give yourself time to allow the suggestions to adhere to your subconscious permanently. Gradually, you will realize the profound effect of your suggestions.

Auto-suggestion for weight loss reinforcement

This exercise will takes only a few minutes to accomplish and should be practiced at least twice a day. You may keep your eyes closed or open. The pauses are indicated by …….. Repeat suggestions when indicated. Never practice this while driving. You may say the following suggestions to yourself quietly or out loud. All it requires is your concentration. If possible, commit these suggestions to memory.

I feel calm….I feel relaxed…..I feel in control……I am calm…..I am relaxed…….I am in control…….I feel safe…….I feel secure……..I'm letting go…….As I let go, all my muscle groups begin to relax…..I feel calm…..I feel relaxed……..I feel in control.

As my muscle groups relax, a beam of sunlight enters my body…..It rids me of all negative thoughts and feelings…..leaving me with only positive thoughts and positive feelings. I feel calm…..I feel relaxed………I am in control.

My subconscious mind is now open to receive the helpful and beneficial suggestions I'm about to give to myself. I feel good about my commitment to take off 1 1/2 - 2 lbs. each week, (repeat this three times). Overeating is very unhealthy to my body (repeat three times), I need my body to be healthy so I can live a healthy life…..I am in complete control of my eating habits…….I feel calm…..I feel relaxed…..I feel in control……I am in control….

Now count forward from 1 to 3 and open your eyes.

You feel refreshed, alert and in control.

A SELF REINFORCEMENT SCRIPT #1

This exercise will help you to "let go" and focus in on meaningful suggestions to achieve your goals. It will take only a few minutes to accomplish and should be practiced at least twice a day. You may keep your eyes open or closed. Never practice this while driving You may say the following suggestions mentally to yourself But If possible out loud will be more effective.

Commit these suggestions to memory. your complete concentration and imagination is required. With your permission I will put the suggestions into a sophisticated, custom audio file with subliminals and backgrounds

"I feel calm....I feel relaxed.....I feel in control......I am calm.....I am relaxed.......I am in control.......I feel safe.......I feel secure........I'm letting go........As I let go, all my muscle groups begin to relax.....I feel calm.....I feel relaxed........I feel in control."

As my muscle groups relax, a beam of sunlight enters my body......It rids me of all negative thoughts and feelings.....leaving me with only positive thoughts and positive feelings. "I feel calm.....I feel relaxed"......

My mind is now open to receive the helpful and beneficial suggestions that I am about to give my self.

A SELF REINFORCEMENT SCRIPT #2

This exercise will help you to focus on meaningful suggestions to achieve your goals.
It should be practiced at least twice each day. You may keep your eyes open or closed. Never practice this while you are driving; At first, recite the following suggestions out loud. Commit these suggestions to memory. Then mentally or quietly to yourself. All that is required is your complete concentration.

"I feel calm....I feel relaxed.....I feel in control......I am calm.....I am relaxed.......I am in control.......I feel safe.......I feel secure........I'm letting go.......As I let go, all my muscle groups begin to relax.....I feel calm.....I feel relaxed........I feel in control."

As my muscle groups relax, a soft warm sensation fills my entire body......It rids me of all negative thoughts and feelings.....leaving me with only positive thoughts and positive feelings. "I feel calm......I feel very very relaxed"......

Now, my mind is open to receive the helpful and beneficial suggestions that
I am about to give my self.

CHAPTER FIVE

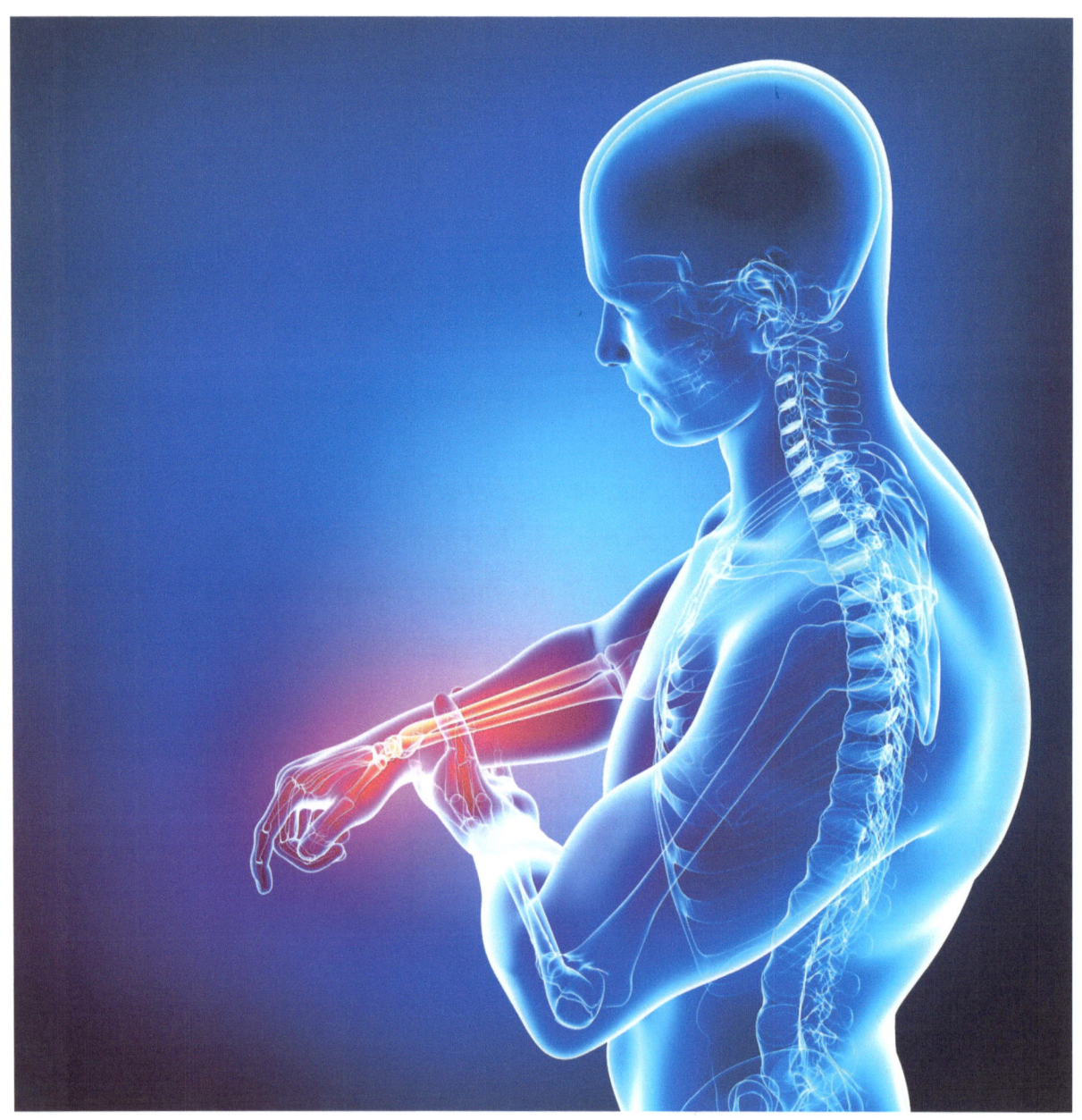

Analgesics, Anesthesia and Controlled bleeding

At depth level 3 level *Analgesia* is possible. The subject would feel no pain,but will experience the sensation of touch.
Level 5 or 6 must be attained for Anesthesia to be experienced with no pain or touch sensations.

Once Anesthesia is attained it is necessary to actively maintain this state, at this level with constant verbal and or other audio reinforcement. Anesthesia is taught at an advanced Level at: www.Anodyne.org

When initiated by a MD or a Dentist It is advisable to use a Hypnotist or a trained assistant transferring the rapport and control to them maintaining the commentary, so that the medical practitioners can concentrate on their task. During surgery it is possible to transfer the rapport to an entire surgical team however obvious problems could ensue if not practiced beforehand in a non critical environment

Maintaining Anesthesia
Auditory Stimuli:
In addition to a prepared script, A Dentist could say-"*As long as you can hear this*-(a computer generated analgesic sound),*You will feel no pain* ".
And or employ all our current technology such as additional Auditory Stimulation, Computer controlled EDMR,Bilateral Rhythm, Psychoactive Tones, and Subliminal audio commands reinforcing the traditional spoken word.

Tactile Stimuli:

The patient can be instructed that *"As long as you keep tapping on the arm rest you will block the pain"*.

The touch of an assistant can act as a surrogate so that the Dentist can concentrate on the dental process.

The patient can be engaged into active participation by instructing them with: "While you are counting backward from 100 you will feel no pain and with each count, you will drift deeper and deeper into a state of *relaxation"*.

Self Hypnosis:

Train a Potential Patient in the use of Self Hypnosis to create their own anesthesia

Combining Hypnosis with Local or General Chemical Anesthesia

Combining Hypnoanesthesia with either a local or a spinal block, during childbirth. Is a very useful modality. The patient will remain conscious, can hear the commentary and respond to a surrogate.

Benefits

With the use of Hypnosis, patients usually require smaller amounts of chemical anesthetic and other drugs. When the patient emerges from anesthesia, Hypnosis can be reintroduced, and suggestions given which to promote more rapid recovery or replace nausea by suggesting,

"You'll be pleasantly hungry". (One cannot perceive hunger and nausea simultaneously).

Hypnosis will greatly reduce recovery time Prior to the infusion of general anesthesia, the use of Hypnosis, can render prior medication for calming unnecessary. Hypnotic suggestions given prior to surgery can lead to more rapid recovery, better cooperation, a more optimistic outlook and can help to minimize bleeding, and possible infection. A shorter stay in the hospital can also be expected.

Today, some hospitals are now using *"Anodyne Imagery" tm*, a registered name for a Hypnotic - pain relief method.

Notes on
HYPNOSIS FOR CONTROLLED BLEEDING

Techniques for bleeding are best studied and practiced with advanced courses such as Anodyne(Tm)

Capillaries: Are the easiest to control with Hypnosis.

Veins: Considered *Medically* impossible, as there are no wall muscles.

Arteries: There is a difference of opinion among the experts.

Some hospitals have effectively used Hypnosis to stop hemorrhaging. With the use of Hypnosis, patients usually require smaller amounts of chemical anesthetic and other drugs. When the patient emerges from anesthesia, Hypnosis can be reintroduced, and suggestions given which to promote more rapid recovery or replace nausea by suggesting,

"You'll be pleasantly hungry".

One cannot perceive hunger and nausea simultaneously

Hypnosis will greatly reduce recovery time

BENEFITS IN CHILDBIRTH

Taught in Advanced courses.

Both to mother and child, with little or no chemical anesthesia, the baby is born much more alert, and in much better shape generally. It is possible for the Mother to see the entire delivery; it's possible to have their eyes open and still maintain anesthesia.

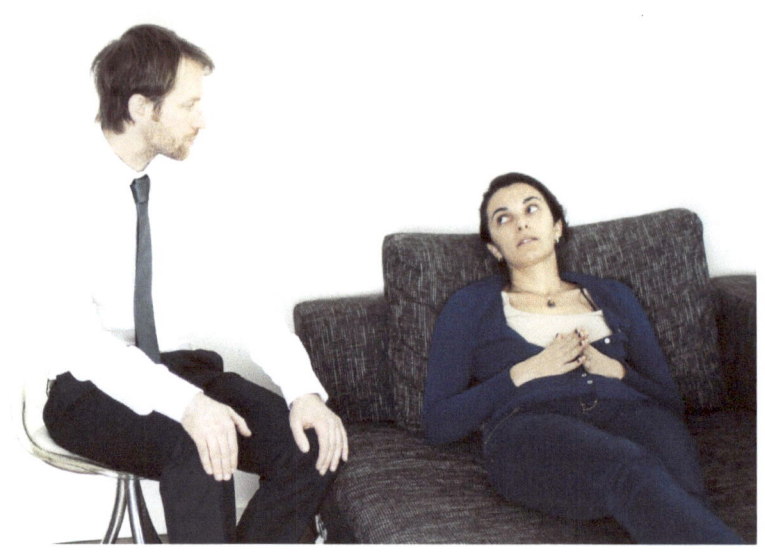

You Are Almost ready To accept the responsibility of your first client's trust.

Implement these practices in an ethical thoughtful manner. You now, are able to install positive and beneficial influences in the life of an individual or yourself. This is very rewarding, but always remember, it is your responsibility to honor the trust granted to you by your clients

Do not apply Hypnosis in circumstances or for conditions in which you are not qualified or if required, to be licensed for under your local laws.

Insurance is necessary, but it can sometimes encourage malpractice issues

Consult with or work under the supervision of a licensed health care professional when applicable

If in doubt refer your client to a licensed health care professional

A First Appointment Template

...............The telephone call or E mail:

Your first statement should be;"How can I help you? Pause and let the caller reply at length or E mail.

If you have determined that your services can be beneficial, explain to the client that the first visits fee will be $XXX.00! And that visit will be essentially a mutual evaluation session including a short "relaxation" Induction.

......This will pre qualify the client financially and their suitably for Hypnosis.

Save any adjustments you may later decide upon for discussion after the first appointment.

It should be without exception,That at the first appointment the first task is to have the client fill out and sign the Consent and Release forms, Medical release documents,if any, a personal data sheet.,and a brief medical history.

Keep digital mutually signed copies in an encrypted,password protected file and give the client the originals.

Give the client a brief qualifying introduction, and initiate a process of rapport, discussing their goals and dispelling any misconceptions by describing Modern, Ethical Hypnosis and that the first session is to be simply "A Guided Relaxation" and how subsequent Modern Ethical Hypnosis sessions can help them to archive their goals

The first session ,and in Subsequent more complex sessions as well,you can use a professionally prepared script using SHARM software in the *record session* mode using your headset/microphone and provide the client as well as possibly an observer,friend or family member sound isolating headsets. With your headset/microphone,you can address the client by name and at your predetermined stages of each session, add your suggestions and personalizations.

After Every session,:

Immediately after bringing the client out of Hypnosis ,enter into a generalized conversation regarding their experience guiding the discussion toward their description of physical and emotional sensations,their concept of time elapsed,and their heart rate. Reinforce the suggestions with oblique positive comments such as "not smoking is having a noticeable effect on your "......." ability or performance! This is a very important and useful part of every session as the subject is still in a receptive state for reinforcement.

CONCLUSION

The exam contained in this course is self administered.

First – You have Taken the exam *Before* reading the manual

You have read the manual, and completed each end of chapter quiz and assignment

Now..Take the exam with the book *open*. Grade yourself, With the enclosed key

Wait one day

Take the Exam again with the Course Manual *closed.*
Grade yourself With the Key.

If you answered 40 out of the 50 questions in the Third Exam Correctly, Make arrangements and payment for an oral interview and and your live session demonstration at the Florida Holistics Institute. The examiner will provide a random subject and evaluate your demonstration to determine that that you can successfully induce the receptive state in a subject.

The examiner will submit a written report with recommendation that the Florida Holistics Institute issue a Certified statement of demonstrated competency and a Certificate.

Henry L. Silvia

Henry L Silvia MCH PhD
Director Florida Holistics Institute

Hardware-Office

Telephone

PC Computer with a minimum of 4gb of RAM, and 1 TB hard drive

A combination Ink-jet Printer, Scanner, Fax. Machine

A separate independent Backup Hard Drive...To Encrypt and store the Client's files and recorded sessions.

A second large, (at least 36in.) Monitor. Wall Mounted for the subject to view when video subliminals are used.

Headsets

For the Operator, The GE #98971 Is a lightweight wired, headset/microphone
The most inexpensive, but high quality combination found after years of selections

Two Sony MDR,985R wireless headsets For sound isolation, and input from computer generated audio files. The One For the Client and one sometimes for an observer or student,-
!

Desk 1 office chair

2 soft swiveling client chairs.

Small Coffee table

Bookcase

Secure in desk File storage for Hard copy.

Recommended Software:

_____ *Microsoft Office*

Or the *Open Office.org suite which is free and* down-loadable..

_____ *The SHARM 4 (studio) (www.Thesharm.com)* is a complete Program Generator for Professional Therapists.   Who can use the unique pure ambient music to create an effective psycho-acoustic experience for quick and deep Hypnosis trance, Record their own Hypnosis scripts or record live with their clients to provide them with a copy of the audio session for home use.

(Offered at a discount to students of PBHI and with the purchase of this Manual)

  You can create a variety of audio sessions to address issues and goals Reduce stress and anxiety, boost self-confidence, enhance creativity, achieve deep relaxation, increase energy to quit smoking or lose weight—the possibilities for are infinite! SHARM has a Short learning curve.
And a user's Guide and video tutorials to get you started as soon as possible. It has an advanced user interface for easy navigation and clean design created specifically with therapists in mind.

There are 100+ ready-to-use sessions and 160+ prerecorded suggestions, with both male and female voices. included

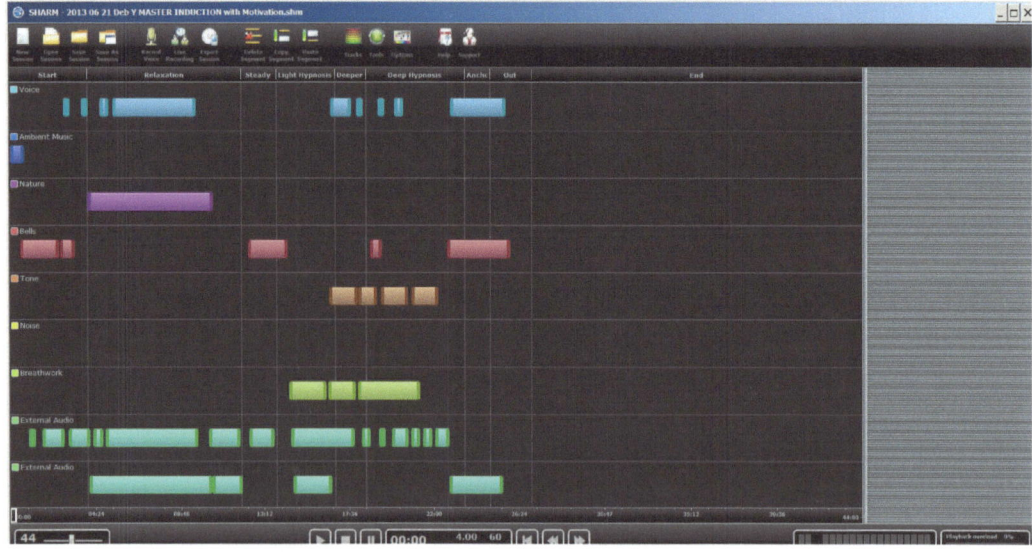

...... software continued

For the advanced students we also include live, hands on demonstration and familiarization for SHARM VISION For **Relaxation and focus** using pure ambient music with Enhanced therapist-client communication to
Immerse your client in a virtual audio scene, in which you can hear each other's voice amidst the music and sounds mixed in the background.

In Clinic, We also use and teach an "off label application" of software that monitors brain activity
There are various choices, we recommend the simplest available as our purpose is simply to detect a "reaction or involuntary response to a suggestion or a specific audio visual stimulus.
It must be purchased separately directly from the providers.

Subliminal Video software We teach In clinic, an off label method of using this type of software to create a variety of Visual Subliminal Reinforcements to a Hypnosis session.
It must be purchased from a provider

A Free, versatile, *Digital Audio Editor*...."Audacity" download it @ http://audacity.sourceforge.net

A separate Discreet webcam Is recommended, but **make certain** that the client understands and signs a consent form that each session may be recorded either visually or audibly and that they may have a copy upon request at any time.
At the PBHI we sometimes use the built in HP Media smart webcam built into a HP pavilion dv6 high end Laptop

The Self administered course test:

Take this test **<u>Before reading</u>** the manual
*Take this test with the manual open **<u>After completing</u>** the course*
*Take this test **<u>Again with the manual closed</u>***

1..........After completing this self study one could induce a Hypnotic Trance?..T............F
2..........Useful recorded Hypnosis techniques have been in use since 1750...T............F
3..........Hypnosis is an altered state of consciousness............................T........F
4..........The Foundation for modern Hypnosis is derived from the teachings of Dr. Erickson..T.........F
5..........The Foundation for modern Hypnosis is derived from the studies of Dr. Mesmer .... T............F
6..........Repeated Hypnosis sessions could be described as conditioned response induction..T...........F
7..........Today, Hypnosis is regarded to be the same as Hypnotherapy..T.........F
8........Drug or Alcohol abuse can be treated with Hypnotherapy.............T.......F
9..........Anodyne Imagery is a proprietary modality for pain relief.........T.......F
10........The persistence of an induced response will increase with each session..T..........F
11........Fears or Phobias can be best treated by a Hypnotist................ T.........F
12.......Hypnosis is essentially a derivative of witchcraft........................T.........F
13...The unconscious mind can differentiate between fact and fiction. T.........F

14....... True Hypnosis requires sleep or a loss of consciousness.............. T........ F
15....... Not everyone is capable of entering Hypnosis................................. T...... F
16....... The Higher IQ individuals are the most difficult to Hypnotize.. T....... F
17........ Rapport is an invaluable asset when inducing a hypnotic trance.. T...... F
18........ There are 6 stages of memory.. T...... F
19........ STM is System Trained Memory... T...... F
20........ Episodic Memories are stored as long term.................................. .T..... F
21......... All Hypnosis is self Hypnosis... ...T..... F
22........ This course identifies 5 phases of a hypnosis session................... T..... F
23........ Rapport is not due to emotional dependency upon the operator.. T..... F
24........ HL Silvia described Hypnosis as a non deceptive placebo.............. T..... F
25........ the technique of Pacing was employed by Dr Erickson............ T..... F
26........ Subjects over the age of 80 are the easiest to work with........... T..... F
27........ People allays tell the truth under Hypnosis.................................... T..... F
28........ Anxiety relieving drugs are an aid to Hypnosis................................ T..... F
29....... Properly conducted Hypnotically induced full body catalepsy can be accomplished without risk of muscle strain.. T....... F
30....... In an Emergency, a loud voice is the best and quickest way to awaken a subject... T..... F
31........ Amnesia is experienced in the second level of Hypnosis................ T..... F
32...... Dr. Flowers developed an induction method using Repetition.......... T........ F
33..... The Hypnotic state can be reinforced by informing the subject that they cannot open their eyes until they are told to do so.................... T..... F
34.... The Whiteboard Induction is an induction intensification method.. T.... F
35...... The Most effective Hypnotic suggestions are "replacements"....... T.... F
36...... Simple short sentences are the most effective suggestions.......... T..... F
37...... Subliminal Deepening is a modern enhancement of Hypnosis........... T.... F
38..... Post Hypnosis suggestions are a useful segment of a session.......... T.... F

39. A widely used induction is called Progressive Relaxation..................T...F
40. Subliminal Visual as well as Subliminal Audio suggestions can be employed in the same session..................T..F
41. Hypnosis can induce the release of natural relaxing Endorphins........T....
42. Repeated ingestion of stimulating or sedative chemicals will eventually displace the naturally occurring, automatically released body chemistry..................T...F
43. Hypnotherapy is an effective, stand alone treatment for chemical addictions..................T...F
44. Repeated Reinforcement is necessary for the long term or permanent success of Hypnotic treatment..................T....F
45. Analgesia is possible at depth level 1..................T....F
46. Capillary bleeding can be controlled with Hypnosis..................T....F
47. It is possible to effectively combine Hypnoanestesia with chemical Anesthesia..................T.....F
48. Most jurisdictions lack any effective licensing requirements regarding Hypnosis..................T...F
49. Subliminal reinforcement has been documented to increase the success percentage of hypnosis for smoking cessation by 500%..................T......F
50. A subject under hypnosis will perform any act commanded by the operator..................T...F

KEY

The Self administered course test

1.........After completing this self study one could induce a Hypnotic Trance?...T.
2....Useful recorded Hypnosis techniques have been in use since ...1750..T..
3..........Hypnosis is an altered state of conciousness......................................T..
4..........The Foundation for modern Hypnosis is derived from the teachings of Dr. Erickson...T..
5..........The Foundation for modern Hypnosis is derived from the studies of Dr. Mesmer ....F....
6..........Repeated Hypnosis sessions could be described as conditioned response induction...T....
7..........Today, Hypnosis is regarded to be the same as Hypnotherapy..........F..
8..........Drug or Alcohol abuse can be treated with Hypnotherapy................T...
9..........Anodyne Imagery is a proprietary modality for pain relief...............T..
10........The persistence of an induced response will increase with each session...T..
11....Fears or Phobias can best be treated by an unsupervised Hypnotist....F..
12.......Hypnosis is essentially a derivative of witchcraft............................F..
13.......The unconscious mind can differentiate between fact and fiction.....F..
14.......True Hypnosis requires sleep or a loss of consciousness....................F..
15.......Not everyone is capable of entering Hypnosis..F..
16.......The Higher IQ individuals are the most difficult to Hypnotize..........F..
17........Rapport is an invaluable asset when inducing a Hypnotic trance........T..
18........There are 6 stages of memory...F..
19........STM is System Trained Memory..F..
20........Episodic Memories are stored as long term................................ ....T..
21.........All Hypnosis is self Hypnosis..T..

22........This course identifies 5 phases of a hypnosis session........................T..
23........Rapport is not due to emotional dependency upon the operator........T..
24........HL Silvia described Hypnosis as a non deceptive placebo....................F..
25..The technique of Pacing was employed by Dr Erickson............................T..
26........Subjects over the age of 80 are the easiest to work with................F.
27........People allays tell the truth under Hypnosis...F.
28........Anxiety relieving drugs are an aid to Hypnosis..T.
29.......Properly conducted Hypnotically induced full body catalepsy can be accomplished without risk of muscle strain...F..
30........In an Emergency, a loud voice is the best and quickest way to awaken a subject..F..
31.......Amnesia is experienced in the second level of Hypnosis........................F.
32......Dr. Flowers developed an induction method using Repetition...............T..
33.....The Hypnotic state can be reinforced by informing the subject that they cannot open their eyes until they are told to do so.........................T..
34....The Whiteboard Induction is an induction intensification method........T..
35......The Most effective Hypnotic suggestions are "replacements"............T..
36......Simple short sentences are the most effective suggestions................T..
37......Subliminal Deepening is a modern enhancement of Hypnosis................T..
38.....Post Hypnosis suggestions are a useful segment of a session...............T.
39..A widely used induction is called Progressive Relaxation.......................'T..
40.....Subliminal Visual as well as Subliminal Audio suggestions can be employed in the same session..T.
41.....Hypnosis can induce the release of natural relaxing Endomorphins.......T.
42....Repeated ingestion of stimulating or sedative chemicals will eventually displace the naturally occurring, automatically released body chemistry....T..

43....Hypnotherapy is effective, when simultaneously applied with treatment for chemical addictions..T..

44....Repeated Reinforcement is necessary for the long term or permanent success of Hypnotic treatment...T..

45.....Analgesia is possible at depth level 1...F..

46.....Capillary bleeding can be controlled with Hypnosis.............................T..

47.....It is possible to effectively combine Hypnoanestesia with chemical Anesthesia..T.

48.....Many jurisdictions lack any effective licensing requirements regarding Hypnosis..T..

49...Subliminal reinforcement has been documented to increase the success rate of Hypnosis for smoking cessation by 500%...T..

50....A subject under Hypnosis will perform any act commanded by the operator...F..

xx

APPENDIX

Forms:

Client Agreement/Consent..................123

Client Intake...124

Stop Smoking agreement....................125

Confidential Suggestions.....................126

Informed Consent 1..............................127

Informed Consent 2..............................128

Primary Session comments..................130

Session operator's comments.............129

1st Session checklist............................130

CLIENT AGREEMENT AND CONDITIONS

For warranty purposes, I agree to follow all suggestions given to me by

_____, or legitimate qualified associates _____ , in the course of our consultation sessions, including the keeping of all scheduled appointments. I understand that if I do not keep my appointments and follow all suggestions given me, we cannot and will not warranty these services without my full cooperation.

I understand that _____ its legitimate qualified associates do not prescribe drugs, diagnose any medical conditions or provide unsupervised treatment for such conditions.

_____ or its legitimate qualified associates, does not practice Mental Health Therapy or provide Medical advice or Treatment.

The methods used are Hypnosis, Visualization, Guided Imagery and Relaxation. (V68.20)

I understand and agree to any recording that or its legitimate qualified associates , may deem necessary during this and future consultations.

I agree to pay for services when rendered, unless other arrangements, in writing are agreed to in advance.

I understand and agree that an appointment canceled or broken without 24 hour advance notice will be charged to me, the client at 1/2 the customary rate.

XXXXXX XXXXXXX, ………………………. Date…………………………………………..

……………………………. Associate……… Date……………………………………..

Client Printed Name………………………………………….

Client....Signature..
Date...

Client Intake Form

Name……………………………………………

Mail Address:……………………………………… Credit

card Type/and#……………………………… ………………… Exp. Date………….

Credit card Security#………. DOB……..

Email…………………………………………

.Telephone…………………………………….

Client's stated Purpose/

Issue v68.20 Non Medical (Y) General

Health statements and declared medications………….

MD/ referral /consulted? (Y)   (NO)

Hobbies/Activities/Interests……..

Education Level/…………/Specialization……

Other Comments, or Information from Client's **Signature** ………………….…**Today's Date**……….

STOP SMOKING AGREEMENT TERMS AND CONDITIONS

For warranty purposes, I agree to follow all suggestions given to me by _____, in the course of our consultation sessions, including the keeping of all scheduled appointments. I understand that if I do not keep my appointments and follow all suggestions given me,_____cannot and will not warranty these services without my full cooperation.

The methods used are Hypnosis, Visualization, Guided Imagery and Relaxation. (V68.20) I understand that _____ does not prescribe drugs, diagnose any medical conditions or provide treatment for such conditions. _____does not practice Mental Health Therapy or provide Medical advice or Treatment.I agree to participate in 5 consecutive Hypnosis Sessions To become an Ex-Smoker.

1. Any time that I may think about a cigarette, I will first take 6 rapid Deep Breaths and then activate my Self-Hypnosis Auto Suggestion to trigger a feeling of deep relaxation and well being.

2. *I will walk 15 minutes every day for the next 30 days*

3. *For the 30 days following my last session, Every Morning, Noon and Evening before going to sleep, I will listen to the audio reinforcement provided on either my own appliances or equipment provided by _____.*

4. *I will increase my intake of water to a minimum of 1 quart per day, consciously seek and consume more fresh fruit, than I normally consume, take supplemental vitamin C with D, and reduce (preferably eliminate) my coffee and alcohol intake.*

5. I understand and agree to any recording that _____or its legitimate qualified associates , may deem necessary during this and future consultations.

6. I agree to pay for services when rendered, unless other arrangements, in writing are agreed to in advance.

7. I understand and agree that an appointment canceled or broken without 24 hour advance notice will be charged to me, the client at 1/2 the customary rate x_____

guarantees his services for the life of the client or for the life of his practice, whichever comes first, providing you, the client have followed all beneficial suggestions and has kept all appointments as agreed., to the extent that You the client, can return for the complete 5 day series at no charge y This applies only for the subject matter of our original consultation and that a period of 30 days have passed since the last consultation.

_____.. Date............ .

Client's Printed Name.. Client's Signature..Date………..

Confidential

Suggestions

Client #..

Suggestion #1

Suggestion #2

Suggestion #3

Informed Consent (non therapeutic Hypnosis)-1

:

Please print your name in the first space, then sign, print and date below to indicate that you understand

That which you have read.

I, _____, agree to engage in the process on non-therapeutic hypnosis. I understand that I will have all choices at all times and can start and end the process at any time. The services Rendered are held out to the public as non-therapeutic hypnotism, defined as the use of hypnosis to inculcate positive thinking and the capacity for self-hypnosis. The services Rendered

are not any form of health care or psychotherapy, and I expect no health benefits. I agree to continue medication as prescribed by my attending and consulting physicians and Licensed Health care providers I understand that hypnotherapy is not a substitute for medical care.

. In the event of a medical emergency or if I feel suicidal, I will I agree to seek medical attention or

call 911 or other emergency help.

I understand that the methods of hypnosis

Include relaxation, deep breathing, creative visualization and other techniques and may produce physical

and emotional responses. I have been informed as to the limits of hypnosis effectiveness and have been offered referral to other providers I also give consent to have all session's reordered by audio/ video or both. I am over age 18, and consent to hypnosis services offered by or Qualified_associates _of_

Signature: _____

Print Name: _____ Date:

Informed Consent (non-therapeutic Hypnosis)-2

Please print your name in the first space, then sign, print and date below to indicate that you understand what you have read.

I, _____ agree to engage in the process on non-therapeutic hypnosis. I understand that I will have all choices at all times and can start and end the process at any time. The services rendered are held out to the public as non-therapeutic hypnotism, defined as the use of hypnosis to inculcate positive thinking and the capacity for self-hypnosis. The services rendered are not represented as any form of health care or psychotherapy, and despite research to the contrary, by law _____ may make no health benefit claims for services rendered. I agree to continue medication as prescribed by my attending physicians and understand that hypnotherapy is not a substitute for medical care. If my symptoms I agree to seek medical attention. In the event of a medical emergency or if I feel suicidal, I will call 911 or other emergency help. I understand that the methods of hypnosis Include relaxation, deep breathing, creative visualization and other techniques and may produce physical and emotional responses. I have been informed as to the limits of hypnosis effectiveness and offered referral to other providers I also give consent to have all session's recorder by audio/ video or both. I am

over age 18, and consent to hypnosis services offered by

_____

Signature: _____

Print Name: _____

Date: _____

Session Operator's Comments:

1ˢᵗ Session Date_____
Subsequent Session dates_____

No Smoking series
 Steps:

Pre-Talk x

Rapport rating_____

Modeling, Mirroring and Pacing Effectiveness_____

Induction Technique used_____

Indirect Methods during rapport_____

Whiteboard Induction _____Y/N

 Deepening Modalities_____

Hypnotic Suggestions List_____

Post Hypnotic List_____

De-Hypnotize-by Operative Active?_ interactive ?_____ Subject's Initiative__?

Commentary/Summary Recommendations to Client:_____

www.ingramcontent.com/pod-product-compliance
Lightning Source LLC
Chambersburg PA
CBHW050719180526
45159CB00003B/1076